# THE
# SECRET
# LIVES OF
# MEN

## What Men Want
## You To Know
## About Love, Sex,
## and Relationships

Christopher Blazina, Ph.D.

**Health Communications, Inc.**
**Deerfield Beach, Florida**

*www.hcibooks.com*

**Library of Congress Cataloging-in-Publication Data**

Blazina, Chris.

The secret lives of men : what men want you to know about love, sex, and relationships / Chris Blazina.

p. cm.

Includes index.

ISBN-13: 978-0-7573-0660-0 (trade paper)

ISBN-10: 0-7573-0660-8 (trade paper)

1. Men—Psychology.  2. Men—Sexual behavior.  I. Title.

HQ1090.B548 2008

155.6'32—dc22

2008033952

Publisher: Health Communications, Inc.
3201 S.W. 15th Street
Deerfield Beach, FL 33442-8190

Cover design by Justin Rothkowitz
Interior design and formatting by Dawn Von Strolley Grove

*For the good folks, past and present,*
*who have taught me to be a guardian for others and myself.*
*To my dad: The first of many to start me down that path.*
*And*
*for Sadie*

# ACKNOWLEDGMENTS

M any thanks to my good friends and colleagues, without whose support this project would have never come to fruition. Each played a pivotal role at various points in this journey: Ed Willems, Dov Liberman, Stewart & Angela Pisecco, Trevor Andrews, Marcy Posner, Lauren Hoffer, Steve Trotter, Mark Hunter, Michele Matrisciani, and Lora Schoen.

# CONTENTS

# INTRODUCTION

In 1949, Arthur Miller's play *Death of a Salesman* debuted. The play is the story of a man who concludes that he is worth more to his family dead than alive. After a lifetime on the road as a traveling salesman, he commits suicide so his family can cash in his insurance policy. Initial reviews of the play noted that many men in the audience were openly crying, a rather unusual occurrence for the time. On the other hand, women seemed somewhat confused, not sure of what to make of the play or exactly why men where so moved by it. Miller's play had revealed a portion of the secret lives of men.

Fifty years later, on the popular TV show *Friends*, Bruce Willis appeared as a special guest star in a role as Rachel's love interest. A familiar relationship pattern emerged in a scene where Rachel asks Willis's tough-guy character to show more of his vulnerable side; to her shock, he does. Willis's character pours out his soul in stories of pain and conflict. Although Rachel gets exactly what she wants—for her boyfriend to open up in a very real way—her response is to feel embarrassed, uncomfortable, and to quickly lose respect for him. Comic relief covers up this portion of the secret lives of men.

Both of these examples highlight portions of the inner world of men that have been exemplified in music, literature, theater, and comedy for centuries. So why is it that our culture systematically trains men from a young age to distance themselves from any vulnerable or emotional aspects of their psyches? This cultural training is not newsworthy in and of itself. As a society, we have gained insight into the sometimes unhealthy but "normal" or "expected" ways that males learn to be men and the "actions" that we determine are "only what a man would do/say." What *is* worth noting is that men really do want to be understood, not cast aside as unemotional, backward thinking, desensitized, or "clueless"—and they desire to connect with others. Men have secret lives, and they are complex and multidimensional.

As a psychology professor, I have taught a course entitled, "Gender Issues in Counseling" at the University of Houston and Tennessee State University. This is usually a small class made up of psychology graduate students working on an advanced degree (master's or PhD), where the women easily outnumber the men, often seven to one. I begin each semester of the course by asking what the students want to learn. They initially give me the "good student" reply, saying that it looked interesting in the course catalog, and they want to apply what they learn to their research or to help the psychotherapy clients they see. Usually, this round of answers lasts for a few minutes, until they look at me and notice I am not buying what they are saying. Then the honest responses come forth, usually in the form of one brave, yet nervous student: "Well, the other reason is . . ."

The other reasons usually involve not understanding men, their fathers, partners, boyfriends, husbands, or sons. Others join in. And from this point on, an open dialogue begins among the mostly female students about how much of a mystery the male psyche is to them and how their taking this class is a proactive way to make their relationships with the men in their lives better. I find that much of what men do seems like a mystery to my female students, and they seem to hope that the answers lie in some mysterious black box that will be opened over the course of the class.

Both the "Gender Issues in Counseling" course and this book address the complex world of men that is waiting to be discovered by those who are ready to see what lies beneath the surface. This advanced course goes beyond the sweeping generalizations about men (or women) you might encounter in some self-help books. This book attempts to explain some of the more difficult issues that men face. These are concerns that, at some level, men wish women understood more about. Because of their life training, which I refer to as the "Ten Commandments of Growing Up Male," not all men possess the exact words to explain the complexities of their inner lives. Due to this lack of precise communication, one might mistakenly conclude that the secret lives of men have no real depth or intricacy.

What you will discover about men in this book will affect you at various levels in understanding your fathers, friends, husbands, partners, and/or sons. Topics related to men and their manhood, whether with family or friends, can turn heated and passionate. These might include: "Why doesn't he tell me what's on his mind? I am not even sure men have emotions!" "All men seem like nothing more than man-children—is there any way for them to be active fathers and responsive spouses?" "Aren't men and women innately different anyhow?"

The intensity of these moments suggests we have a lot of personal investment in their outcome. Uncovering the inner lives of men can tap into themes of disappointment, frustration, or unfulfilled hopes. I will share some of the stories I have heard from students, clients, friends, and even a few from my own life about these matters, ones that ultimately reflect a deeper complexity about men. The common thread that links all of these case studies is that men want to be better understood and to have better connections with the important people in their lives. Those on the other side of what sometimes feels like a great divide (you, for instance) also want the same. This book serves as a bridge between you and the man you want to know and understand.

As a professor psychologist, I am often asked about my special interest in the field of "men's psychology." I once had a job interview where afterward I was pulled to the side by an older male interviewer who said, "What a relief . . . after reading about all that men's stuff on your résumé, some of us assumed you were gay or something." That "or something" response seems to be a common one initially for those who are trying to understand where my professional interests lie. After all, why would a man study other men? One of the reasons I got into this field of study no doubt had to do with my own upbringing, as I watched my father and men like him struggle with a John Wayne or Frank Sinatra Rat Pack notion of how to be a man. While widely accepted, to me these approaches seemed more like masks that men learned to put on in order to conform to society's notion of the right or appropriate way to be a man.

I have often been privy to a different side of men, one in which they put aside the disguise, showing a more authentic part of themselves. The results have not always been pretty, sophisticated, or relationally skilled by some standards, but when men let their guards down, not expecting a heavy-handed response for being themselves, often something endearing and worth getting to know appears. Accompanying this can be a surprising complexity of emotions and depth of connection. In fact, some of the most influential people in my life who I count on as go-to supports and confidants are men.

On the other side of the coin, women—friends, family, and clients—have confided to me about the pain some men have caused them. Complaints range from the "he is just not that in to me," to "all the good ones are taken," to "can't live with 'em; can't live without 'em." One woman I went out with told me that "if this didn't work out," she was thinking about dating women; not that she was a lesbian or anything, but she figured she had worked through all the viable single men in the local area and was in dire need of fresh company on date night. Sometimes a lack of sensitivity, not being able to talk about any feelings other than sex and anger, or playing the role of a self-absorbed man-child leaves deep scars. Or there is a significant letdown when hope feels extinguished about the possibility of finding a romantic partner who is emotionally mature and sturdy enough to undo some of the old hurts from the past. Growing up with five sisters clued me in about some of these themes at an early age, though I certainly had my own lessons to learn.

I am sympathetic to both sides. Sometimes I even wonder why there has to be sides. While some of the things men and women struggle with may appear very different in terms of content, if you look below the surface there are some remarkable emotional and psychological parallels. After all, men and women are of different genders, not different species. I stress in this book that men and women are more alike than they are different. That notion may seem startling to some. You might even be tempted to put down this book in disbelief.

While it may seem like CNN should have a twenty-four-hour news channel devoted to the latest breaking news about how men and women are different, this line of research has been controversial and inconsistent in findings. There are only a few areas showing reliable differences between men and women, but even these are a matter of controversy. It is not known if they are due to a gender's unique genetic makeup, the differing socialization men and women sometimes experience, or a combination of both. For instance, from preschool forward across the life span, males show higher forms of physical aggression. One might quickly conclude that this is because they have higher levels of testosterone or the male brain is wired differently. However, this finding has to be considered in light of girls showing significantly higher forms of *relational aggression* than boys. That is, they are more likely to resort to indirect forms of aggression to damage the relationships of their peers, by spreading rumors, making fun of them behind their backs, or simply ignoring them.

Research also suggests that the genders may differ in terms of *emotional sensitivity*, or being able to express and then interpret others' emotions. As we will see, there are powerful social forces that shape both men's and women's ability to master these skills. The power of socialization or a painful personal history can sometime make it functional in a sort of dysfunctional way not to know what is going on in your own emotional world. A damaged emotional past may prevent some from fully mastering emotional skills, because to recognize emotions in others usually involves applying the same skills to oneself. Not being good at emotional sensitivity temporarily buffers emotional pain because you are out of touch with what you really feel.

However, it would be inaccurate to conclude that all men (or women for that matter) share the exact characteristics or skill sets. You may be familiar with the statistical notion of the "bell-shaped curve," which pinpoints the exact mathematical average of any attribute within the population at large, but the bell curve also shows the wide variability in the population on any given attribute, from shoe size, to height, to weight. It is a way of categorizing and comparing.

These same notions can be applied to concepts of gender. Keep in mind that the research that purports "differences" between men and women does this usually by using the mathematical average found in the bell curve, so it's making comparisons based on the average man and average woman. Trying to use the "exact" average person as a good representative of everyone within any group, gender or otherwise, may deprive one of a full appreciation for the wide range of people along the continuum who helped form the standard.

Within any gender, there is a range of individuals with various abilities, skills, and talents, and this suggests that a single norm cannot possibly represent everyone in a meaningful way. We have to recognize that there are a variety of men and women who are good—and not so good—at things like emotional sensitivity; otherwise, there wouldn't be successful counselors, psychologists, or caregivers of both genders. Basing research on an "average" by which everyone is compared can lead to sweeping generalizations and stereotypes that are often not accurate and that do not account for exceptions to the average rule on any gender-related differences.

Studies that suggest the average male and female differ in terms of emotional IQ or math and verbal skills lead some to conclude, "Hey, you can't do [fill in the blank], you're a man [or woman]!" We must be careful to guard against letting the research leave us with a skewed view of what men and women are capable of. Given the problems with research on gender differences, some experts within the field of psychology have advocated ending the pursuit of this line of inquiry entirely, focusing instead on the wide range of differences found within each gender; that is, studying the many unique ways men may differ among other men (and likewise for women among women). After all, while cultural expectations may leave a false impression about gender differences, there is not just one way to be a man or a woman.

# The Purpose of This Book

I once heard an interview that the legendary country music singer/songwriter Conway Twitty gave before he died. Someone asked him if he had a particular inspiration when writing his love songs. He said he did; he thought about a guy slow-dancing with his wife. When the song conveyed his feelings for her, which he either could not or would not articulate, he could squeeze her hard, expressing, without the use of his own words, "That's how I feel toward you, honey." In terms of this book, I have a similar mental picture of a caring partner saying to her man, "I don't understand you at all!" and him responding, "Well, if you turn to page 121, you will!" My hope is that whether through Conway Twitty's love songs or some aspects of this book, men will be better understood.

Besides describing the secret lives of men, another aim of this book is to offer guidance for those who wish to help the boys and men they care for. By enacting the role of what I will call a "guardian," both men and women can help a son, partner, father, brother, or friend discover or reorient himself toward his own unique version of being a man. The guardian helps accomplish this task through supplying special types of experiences, such as support, challenge, providing information, clearing up conflicts, and healing past emotional wounds that are specifically related to being a man.

The guardian concept is different from any other approaches found in today's self-help literature for men in that it does not rest upon a foregone conclusion about how men should be ideally defined or enabled. The goal of most self-help books has been to encourage men to follow a set formula or checklist in order to become the ultimate man, according to the given author's spiritual/religious beliefs, social/political agenda, and/or racial/ethnic milieu. But those approaches only push men further into the "proper," cookie-cutter model to which most, if not all, men are pressured to conform.

If the self-help author's approach is well received, it can take on a fadlike quality, and people begin to believe that the ultimate "secret" to real masculinity has been found at last. For the most part, these self-help approaches mean well, but instead of creating lasting guidance for all men, what usually occurs is a "serving" of the flavor of the month regarding manhood for a select few. Those men for whom the latest manhood craze does not ring true are often left feeling even more bewildered and alienated from themselves and others. Rather than presenting another checklist, model, or new fad to follow that men must align with to be "real men," my goal is to show men and their loved ones how to find or reconnect with their authentic selves—a much more difficult and lasting set of skills. Acting as a guardian for a male loved one can help him to do this.

The first chapter, "The Ten Commandments of Growing Up Male," explores the specific socialization many men encounter as they grow up. These guidelines are the ones that men feel are written in stone. From very early on, these commandments guide men's notions of what it means to be a man, and they can often lead to confusion concerning sex and intimacy, make men fearful of anything associated with the feminine, and make them feel there is only one acceptable way to be a man. Understanding the impact that these commandments make can help us to rewrite new commandments. The following are some of the potential benefits of reading and implementing the suggestions in this book:

1. Find out about the *secret shoebox*, the metaphoric place where a man keeps his most intimate thoughts and feelings. Discover what you can do to let a man feel safe enough to unlock that "holy of holies." This can be applied to your boyfriend, husband, brother, son, father, and male friends.

2. Learn how to stand by your man in the ways that he really needs but may be afraid to ask, which will help him, in turn, learn the same for you.

3. Tired of lifeless zombies or frustrating man-children? Imagine instead a mature, grown-up man who is a fully functional, responsive partner, able to be his own man and yours too. Discover what you can do to make this a reality.

4. Have a better sex life with your romantic partner. Communication is a big key. Get on the same page about what feels hot and what does not.

5. Sometimes the legacy of "long ago" still plays a part today; see what can be done to make peace with the pain of the past. This includes resolving issues with parents that still affect his notion of being a man.

6. Gain insight into new approaches to help raise your son. Help is on the way for moms and single moms. Read about a new approach called the "guardian."

7. Besides your husband or son, your dad may be the most important male in your life. Understand that aging can take a toll. See what you can do to help him with that transition.

8. Ever feel frustrated about trying to give feedback to a man? We will learn how to avoid the major relationship land mines and actually let healthy conflict deepen our relationships.

9. Learn practical skills that will help successfully navigate the secret lives of men. This is the advanced course for those interested in a deeper understanding of the inner world of males.

# PART I

# THE SECRET, INNER WORLD OF MEN

# 1

# The Ten Commandments
# of Growing Up Male

We are a rule-driven society. Read some of the great Western philosophers like Rousseau, Locke, or Hobbes, all of whom were very concerned with social contracts that ensured that the powerful did not devour the powerless. Or, on a less cerebral level, rent a copy of the black-and-white version of *The Lord of the Flies*, the film showcasing what happens when a planeload of British schoolboys are stranded on a deserted island with no adult supervision. I will give you a hint: it looks less like *Gilligan's Island* and more like *Survivor* on steroids with an entirely new meaning for being voted off the island.

As a society we shy away from anarchy as a general rule. As a result, there are school rules, religious rules, traffic rules, etiquette rules, work rules, and so on. It is no surprise there are very specific ones that have been created for men—well-established societal messages that males receive about how to be a man—that I have identified as "The Ten Commandments of Growing Up Male." This might conjure up the image of a bearded Moses-like figure descending from the mountain with stone tablets in his hands; a hush falls over the crowd as he declares in a powerful, authoritative voice that these are the commandments for men, laws that all men must follow or punishments will ensue.

For many men, these commandments carry a level of authority that should never be questioned. They are ingrained into our culture as irrefutable truths. Sometimes men who have broken these commandments have received somewhat unsympathetic punishments from a society that can be uninformed about the struggles that men face. Subsequently, there is a trickle-down effect from cultural to familial law, when unwitting parents enforce the commandments through harsh reprimands. While parents think they are helping prepare their sons for the real world through conforming to the commandments, too often a boy's spirit or sense of individualism is broken as a result. These commandments cannot only have powerful effects upon men's emotional and physical well-being, but they also touch the people dear to them. If a boy or man feels weighted down as a result of following the commandments, those in his inner circle can also suffer.

Given the vast number of societal rules that have been created over the years, rest assured that not all of them are good ones; some are outdated, and others need to be rewritten. The same is true for the commandments for men. These societal rules and standards have taken a particular shape over hundreds of years. Greek mythology, the shift from pagan to Christian religion in the Holy Roman Empire, medieval mind-sets and philosophy, misinterpreted scientific research applied to gender roles, folklore, and social tradition are but a few of the cultural dynamics that play a part in shaping how we think men (and women too) should be. Without considering how culture has evolved, and with it expectations for both genders, some might assume things have stayed exactly the same since the cavemen era. As a society we can take many of the previously held truths and run with them, limiting both genders in the process. (For a more extensive discussion on the evolution of masculinity in Western culture, see my previous book, *The Cultural Myth of Masculinity*.)

The astute observer will note that many of these commandments are impossible to keep, even on a man's best day. Some of these are outdated and others are just downright dysfunctional, asking men to be someone they are not. Those of us who have spent our careers studying the secret lives of men have seen how men of all ages are negatively affected by these commandments in both work and love. After all, a man's sense of masculinity affects every avenue of his life. As we talk about each of the commandments, we will address where each one leads men astray.

From the very beginning, I want to stress that the secret lives of boys and men are full of struggles, but it should also be noted that there is the potential for joy and happiness as well. Sometimes men's secret worlds are primal and passionate, while other times they are noble and self-sacrificing. There isn't a "man conspiracy" to keep you distant and confused, and by understanding more about the world of men, you, as a partner, parent, or friend, can learn better ways to give support, gently confront problem areas, and assist a man to be all that he can be. And by the way, these commandments are not set in stone; in reality, they are clay tablets ready to be rewritten—or broken.

# Commandment 1:
### "There is only one way to be a man."

Boys learn from early on that there is a single, right way to be a man. Many of the Commandments for Growing up Male highlight what ideal masculinity looks like. It is usually some variation of an old John Wayne or, more recently, Jason Bourne character: tough, stoic, and self-sufficient. This version of manhood stresses the importance of being powerful and protecting your flanks at all costs. Taken together, all of these characteristics add up to stereotypical masculinity, the singular definition for how all men feel compelled to be.

The notion that there is only one way to be a man is a prime example of the confusing and misleading nature of the commandments. As noted above, research has shown that the definition of "ideal masculinity" has changed over the course of history. Historians who study gender issues have noted that ideal masculinity has it fads and trends just like clothing. Sometimes the ideal man is the tough warrior or cowboy, other times the peace-loving and refined statesman, and still other times, the hard-driving capitalist or the man who goes from rags to riches. For instance, chivalrous knights during the Middle Ages curled their hair and wore tight tunics, pointy shoes, and other eye-catching adornments. Sounds a little like today's metrosexual men, doesn't it? This version of an overstylized man seems to come back into vogue every once in a while throughout the centuries.

Gender historians have also shown that at various points in time there have been multiple, competing notions of what an ideal man looks like. While there may be a singular, most popular version of masculinity, there are still multiple definitions of how to be a man in present society. In fact, scholars claim that there are at least six distinct forms of ideal masculinity operating right now in the United States. That is, there are multiple masculinities based on religion, social class, sexual orientation, political agenda, religion, ethnicity, and race. Even within these broad categories of masculinity, there are still more subfactions, multiplying the number of potential masculinities even further. In fact, we may further stretch this notion and say that there are potentially as many unique ways to be a man as there are different types of individuals. From my perspective, that is exciting news, because it means men may enjoy more freedom to be themselves and really develop their own notion of what it means to be a man.

So the idea that there is only one way to be a man is really off the mark. Boys may be aware of the most popular version of masculinity and conclude, just like their parents, there is only one way to be. They then may feel pressured by society or family to conform to that version, as if pushed through a giant cookie cutter. They feel the demands to do the accepted thing whether it genuinely reflects who they are or not. The consequence of conforming is that men cut away authentic parts of themselves that they determine are not acceptable to the popular version of manhood. In the long run, this has an impact on their ability to be successful at work and love. We will revisit the importance of men being true to themselves later.

# Commandment 2:

## *"Fear the feminine."*

In part, males learn to be men through others telling them what *not* to do. That is the funny thing about learning to be a man; instructions are often heavier on the "don'ts" than the "dos." This is because the rules for being a man are not entirely clear; some of them make no sense, while others are at times contradictory and confusing. However, there is one sure-fire rule that can be counted on: "Don't do anything feminine."

We usually associate the feminine with the world of women; the feminine comes to represent all those inherent aspects that are by their very nature womanly and so surely "not male." So when a man crosses the line into what is perceived as the feminine world, he knows this is a forbidden realm from which he should remove himself as quickly as possible. Historically, the feminine is seen as a corrupting force to masculinity. The worst thing that can be said to a boy is that he is "acting like a girl." I'm not sure who should be more offended: the boy being called a girl or the girl who is being labeled as what not to be!

But what exactly is feminine? Until recently, we could divide the world of emotions, physical or intellectual abilities, and career trajectories along gender lines. For instance, for some time there has existed an unquestioned notion of men's versus women's work. Others believe that men and women are so dissimilar in terms of their emotional needs that they could be from different planets. There are always eye-catching headlines that continue to promote this separatist line of thinking. However, over the last thirty years, these notions, once held as absolute truths, are being reconsidered. Those "masculine" possibilities that society told women they could never attain, like moving up the corporate ladder or obtaining political or professional success, have been revised and/or abandoned. Likewise, men have challenged the notion that being a good parent or partner belongs exclusively to the realm of women. In fact, there has been a 60 percent increase in stay-at-home fathers in the past few years.

While some may see these changes as an erosion of an important distinction between the sexes that results in gender confusion, for me it highlights the truth that some things labeled as a "woman thing" or a "man thing" are really *human* things. We can all participate and be successful in matters of work and love. A man becomes handicapped when he cannot utilize his human skills because they are labeled as feminine ones, and consequently off-limits.

# Commandment 3:
*"Men must funnel all of their feelings into sex or aggression."*

Because men are taught to fear the feminine, they must avoid anything associated with it, and chief among these aspects are emotions. From the formative years onward, boys are placed into a bind because the emotional aspects inherited as a part of their natural birthright are deemed off-limits. Along the way, the commandment about fearing the feminine takes hold, and they learn that emotions are bad things. People might make fun of men for showing things like sensitivity, vulnerability, and tenderness; these traits are seen as aspects that corrupt a man's sense of masculinity. As a result, many men learn to keep their emotions in check. Or, worse yet, they don't allow themselves to experience feelings *at all*, and after utilizing this coping skill for thirty or forty years, some of them end up in the emergency room, thinking they have had a heart attack. The ER physician might explain that they have just had a panic attack and should go speak to someone about the pent-up stress they are carrying.

Emotions are hardwired human parts, and we all have them, but men learn in their "man-training" to cope with them in ways that are consistent with the commandments. Men feel compelled to mask them, funneling their entire emotional range into two socially acceptable "male" emotions: sex and aggression. These traits, which can disguise other, more vulnerable, off-limits feelings, allow men to maintain a tough exterior. In short, sex and aggression are the quintessential male emotions. What can appear as a stunted emotional repertoire often gives the impression that men are emotionally devoid of real feelings, or at best, that they are simple creatures who are only concerned with primal matters. But we will see later that even with this masking of emotions, a man's feeling function is still multidimensional and complex. The emotional realm of the secret lives of men is complicated, and we will spend time sorting through it.

# Commandment 4:
*"Affection is always associated with sex."*

We begin to see how some commandments are interrelated. If you fear the feminine, it has a direct effect upon how you express feelings in the form of sex or aggression, which in turn skews the definitions, limitations, and boundaries of some emotions. A prime example of this is that men are taught early on that emotional intimacy is interchangeable with physical intimacy. So if you feel close to someone, it means you also want to have sex with them. This misunderstanding about emotional and physical intimacy causes lots of trouble. It can lead to some complicated questions for men and women, such as can men and women be "just" friends? From this perspective, they can't, because if a man grows emotionally close, sexual feelings are inevitable (at least from the man-training perspective).

This fallacy about tender feelings always equaling sexual ones also affects the closeness between two good male friends; after all, the same formula is present. This makes men uncomfortable about getting too close and stirs up homophobic reactions. Many straight men try to circumvent this issue when they get together so that any ensuing emotional intimacy can be explained away through drinking too much or through the joy of playing sports together, where hugs or pats on the butt are just a part of the game. Men are invited at many points in their lives to rethink these issues and see with clearer eyes that love and sex are not always synonymous.

# Commandment 5:

*"You big ape: boy society is based on power, strength, and paranoia."*

Boys grow up in a culture that stresses the outward appearance of strength and power. Young men feel compelled to jockey for position on the social ladder as if they are in some Darwinian survival of the fittest. This male hierarchy is based on how well a boy can adhere to the commandments. If he is successful, he can earn masculine currency to put in the bank. And what does he think can be purchased with this big man's bank account? Well, just about anything he wants: a beautiful wife, more power and success, eternal youth, and everlasting happiness. Confirmation of the "more masculine currency = lasting happiness" equation seems pervasive. After all, look at movie stars and professional athletes—they are all happy, aren't they? But let's say, for instance, that a man doesn't measure up to the commandments—what then?

The legacy of the big ape mentality can affect a man's (boy or grown-up) life expectations and his ability to secure a mate or have a chance at long-term success or happiness. This is one of the reasons men feel especially emotionally walloped when they lose their job: they imagine that someone has made a run on the bank and drained all their man-currency from their account. What do they do now? Who would be willing to love them? One of the struggles men face is learning they are more than the adolescent version of masculinity that was presented to them when they were growing up and that their virtue as a man is not entirely tied to being the biggest, most fierce ape on the block.

Another offshoot of this misguided big ape mentality is that a man becomes more of a man by taking from others. In fact, some have argued that this process is a rite of passage that ushers in manhood. This applies to all manner of things, like seizing someone else's property, wealth, significant other, and self-esteem. Built into this rather off-balance way of growing up is an understandable level of paranoia. Men learn to never show their vulnerable side and always give the impression they are in control, so as to fend off potential attacks. If others smell his inferiority or weakness, they will surely be ready to pounce. We will look at how this level of suspicion erects barriers that affect all forms of intimacy.

Another troubling aspect of the big ape mentality is the sheer futility of being able to sustain that bulletproof pose. Even men who are more naturally inclined toward the commandments cannot keep them all. Researchers note that keeping all the expected, traditional rules of being a man is like walking a tightrope that literally no one can stay on; what ensues is something referred to as "male gender role conflict," the psychological strain related to being a man. In fact, gender role conflict, which has been explored for more than twenty years, is associated with a wide assortment of problems, such as increases in depression, anxiety, substance abuse, and various interpersonal problems. Male gender role conflict has even been found in boys, creating a similar psychological strain for them. This suggests that the man-making process can have a cumulative effect, one that weighs heavily on boys and men.

It is not a matter of *if* a man will stumble and fall in regards to traditional expectations, but *when* and *how many times* a day. So a man will feel compelled to cover up his shortcomings through the use of *man defenses* and coping skills. One of the tools men use in moments of vulnerability—moving toward others in an aggressive way—is learned in boyhood. Man defenses can involve brutality, displacing pain onto others, or emotional and physical withdrawal. Boys are not the only ones who utilize these skills; when grown men find themselves in moments of uncomfortable, interpersonal vulnerability or evaluation, they are prone to make use of their old defenses. Feeling they are under the microscope pushes men into what seems like a dangerous space. This makes receiving legitimate feedback from wives or bosses difficult. More in-depth ideas about how to give constructive feedback will be given later in the book.

# Commandment 6:

*"A boy needs a male role model or his sense of being a man is flawed."*

The idea that a boy must have a male role model is deeply embedded in the cultural lore, which says that boys learn how to be men by cutting ties with mom and imitating a grown man. The adult male gives the boy instructions for what is proper and improper behavior based on the commandments and, in particular, with regards to fearing the feminine. The male role model is seen as a sort of initiator who turns the boy into a man. This model of making boys into men is so well accepted that it has become the stuff of TV holiday melodrama and primetime sitcoms. Even when it is presented as a satire, it still reflects the culturally accepted premise that boys can only learn about manhood through the successful tutelage of a male role model. If he does not have this experience, he is presumed lost.

While the potential for disaster in using this model for forming men can make the Homer Simpsons of the world nervous, many moms are apprehensive of it as well. Wives worry that their husbands or other potential male role models are too distant physically or emotionally to provide this training. And what about Mom? Is she supposed to help in some way with her son's journey to manhood? After all, she has no doubt been exposed to men's fear of the feminine and wonders if her presence really is corrupting to her son's sense of masculinity.

We will look at some of the shortcomings of the male role model idea later, including the idea that forcing someone to imitate another person's version of masculinity does not help a male of any age find his own authentic notion of being a man. In lieu of the male role model approach, we will talk about a new perspective for helping boys and grown men. This is based on the idea that all males need *guardians*; guardians can be of either gender and are invested in males developing into their own sense of being a man, not imitating someone else's version. After all, that is what we should value the most about our man: his ability to be himself.

# Commandment 7:

*"If your father is rejecting, you must learn to please him."*

While the male role model theory is fraught with potential liabilities, there is another part of the man-making equation that deeply affects males. One of the most difficult legacies involves a boy who did not receive his father's blessing; that is, a boy who did not feel affirmed as a "good man" by his father (or father figure). In cultural lore, the father is the prototypical male, carrying the most significance. A boy may learn skills from a male role model who is not his family member, but his father is the ultimate source of masculinity.

Many men carry painful memories of not living up to their father's expectations, most of which are somehow related to not keeping the commandments. Men may feel they disappointed their father figure, and because of this, his approval was withheld. There may be specific messages about what needs to be done regarding achievements or behaviors before the father can give his blessing. When this scenario is played out, it can seriously affect the father/son relationship, resulting in hostility, hurt, or emotional coldness. The specific repercussions upon the unblessed son are that he feels incomplete and unworthy.

Many men wonder what is wrong with them; what tragic unlovable flaw do they carry that their father could not or would not bless them as a good man? The son concludes he is not worthy of love, respect, or care. Sadly, even if the son has many others around him who see the good in him and let him know it, his father's perceived disapproval can trump them all. He continues to operate in that frozen little-boy mode of thinking, looking to see if this latest round of accomplishments finally brings him up to snuff.

The hard work that many of these sons need to do involves getting to know their fathers as real people beyond the role of parent. This will open their eyes in a compassionate way to the notion that their fathers also have their own hang-ups and conflicts about being men. The commandments affect each age-group, and tragically, the pain from one generation of men is often passed on to the next. If a man's father carries his own wounds, this has no doubt impacted his ability to give the blessing his son deserved; it had nothing to do with the son's worth as a man. In fact, often a father unwittingly tries to make his son a better man in the areas in which he himself falls short. Depending on the father's own level of conflict in these matters, it can sometimes lead to over-the-top reactions when he sees his son following in his footsteps. The deeper spirit of helping his son "do better" can originate from a good place but can come across in damaging ways. Later, we will explore how sons of all ages may have to deal with this issue, grieve, and make peace with the "father wound."

# Commandment 8:

*"If you don't please your mother, you must marry someone like her."*

The smothering mother is another idea built into cultural lore. It usually conjures up an image of boys tied to mom's apron strings. However, if we look closely, this smothering is not really gender-specific and can occur with either parent. It involves a caregiver who is unable to keep his or her own needs and biases in check when it comes to the son. Smothering is really about squelching a budding sense of individualism and authenticity. This can take a number of forms, and one stereotypical version involves a boy being lulled into a rather unhealthy relationship with his mother. Because of unfinished work on the mom's part, including not having an emotionally fulfilling relationship with her romantic partner, she may turn to her son to help with the empty feelings and loneliness. Mothers with smothering issues dress their boys up as the little man they always wanted but never had. They elevate them from the status of son to emotional partner. Moms confide in and depend on them in ways that are not appropriate. Some may even be more than a bit jealous when their boy begins to take note of other girls.

This is a destructive arrangement for everyone involved. The ultimate outcome of the situation is that both the son and the mother will remain emotionally unfulfilled. The son cannot really assume the role that the mom needs and is left with an emotional legacy. He may feel angry or put upon when he thinks about his relationship with his mother. There may be struggles to put distance between him and her so he can live his own life. Some of this may follow him into adulthood. You would think that when he comes of age and begins looking for a romantic partner, he would run from anyone bearing the slightest resemblance to a smothering caregiver, but sometimes the exact opposite happens. He chooses someone who also has some smothering tendencies—not because he is a glutton for punishment but because it is what is most familiar to him, what he is comfortable with in an uncomfortable way. In other words, he has unfinished psychological and emotional work to do that centers on his own worth as a man. The unconscious hope is that by replaying old scenarios with new people, there will be a different outcome. In this case, he wishes to be in a loving relationship without the risk of losing his sense of identity. We will look at the legacy of a son's relationship with his caregivers and how it can unwittingly guide men in many avenues of their lives.

# Commandment 9:
### *"Being a man is a 24/7 job."*

Researchers have noted that trying to fulfill all the duties related to being a man can become a strong preoccupation. One of the difficult things to appreciate is that being a man is a 24/7 job. You really are never off duty, and you're always on call. A man never knows when someone or something will ask him to account for his manliness. When this happens, he can't say, "Well, I think I will take a holiday from being a man today." Not only is he taught the stringent rules for being a man, but he must follow them at all times.

The closest thing a man gets to a break from the commandments is when he is sick. I am sure you know the widely held impression about tough men acting like babies when they are under the weather. Colleagues may look at them in disbelief and say, "What is wrong with Sonny today? He looked kind of misty and told me how much he really valued our friendship . . ." "Well, he has been sick lately; must be that bird flu going around." For a man to deviate from the commandments, he needs a written doctor's excuse. When a man is given the social nod of approval to show off-limit parts of himself, like vulnerable emotions or neediness, there is usually a flash-flood event; after all, these natural parts of being human have been pent-up for a long time.

Added to this burden of constant self-scrutiny about measuring up to the commandments is making sure that others (and sometimes oneself) are not aware of any shortcomings. Much effort and work is invested in keeping all of this stuff hidden from view. Sometimes I ask male clients to envision what they would do with all the leftover emotional and psychic energy if they were not so preoccupied with adhering to the commandments. I often see a light go on in their eyes as their imaginations run wild. They could get to the novel they always wanted to write, really connect with their partner and kids, or finally chart a course that feels authentic and rewarding. If you are a partner or wife, you might also feel this same exciting jolt at the prospect of your man having more freed-up resources. This may transcend the ultimate "Honey-do list" where his surplus of energy moves beyond finally cleaning out the gutters or sometimes watching the kids to entering into a new phase of life where he is able to connect with you in ways thought impossible before. Everyone benefits when a man finds peace with the commandments.

# Commandment 10:

### "A man must follow the commandments even if it causes him to be emotionally stunted or leads him off track."

The commandments can leave many men at risk for becoming emotionally stunted or simply lost. I have discussed elsewhere the notion of the

"fragile masculine self"; this is when men miss out on the emotional sustenance needed to become their own unique person and instead carry a sense
of brokenness inside they feel compelled to hide even from their closest
relations. As noted in a previous section, the strains related to being a man
(i.e., male gender role conflict) have been charted for some time and reflect
serious troubles.

However, recent research suggests that men begin to feel the brunt of
male socialization as boys. Starting in the formative years, a man learns to
bend himself to others' whims, which gets him off track in terms of being
his own man. The values that should form the basis for his core sense of
identity and be a source of strength throughout his life instead get misplaced or mislabeled and cast aside. When a partner, parent, or friend asks
who he really is, he might have more success describing the persona he
feels pressured to assume rather the actual makeup of his own internal
world and values.

It is ironic that one of the things society values most is a man who has his
own unique style and sense of individualism, yet the commandments can
actually separate him from that foundational aspect of who he is. Men are
taught to conform at all costs instead of becoming their own healthy versions of what it means to be a man. Unfortunately, we have been grappling
in the dark for a while now, trying to come up with a one-size-fits-all version
of masculinity. Many pop psychology books will tell you otherwise, but the
truth is, there isn't such a thing. As long as we ask men to adjust to the
newest and latest fad of masculinity, they will continue to be lost to themselves and to those they love.

I'm offering a different and subsequently more difficult path, a tailor-
made version of masculinity based on who a man actually is—his genuine
values, disposition, and character—in short, his true sense of self. Let's stop
asking all men to fit into a size forty-two regular. Instead, we can value a
man for finding his own healthy fit and style; this in turn will help propel
him on to success and contentment in both work and love. Instead of lifeless zombies or frustrating man-children, imagine a mature, grown-up man

who is a fully functional, responsive partner, able to be his own man and yours too. If you are reading this book, no doubt you have a vested interest in this outcome. By helping your man find his way, you will enrich your life as well. While a man must ultimately do this work himself, this book is a guide to assist you in the process. Welcome to the secret lives of men.

## "The Commandments of Growing Up Male"

---

1. There is only one way to be a man.

2. Fear the feminine.

3. Men must funnel all of their feelings into sex or aggression.

4. Affection is always associated with sex.

5. You big ape: boy society is based on power, strength, and paranoia.

6. A boy needs a male role model or his sense of being a man is flawed.

7. If your father is rejecting, you must learn to please him.

8. If you don't please your mother, you must marry someone like her.

9. Being a man is a 24/7 job.

10. A man must follow the commandments even if it causes him to be emotionally stunted or leads him off track.

---

## ▶ Toolbox Tip: Challenging the Commandments

The astute observer may notice that many of the commandments are interlocked and interrelated. For instance, the second commandment, "Fear the feminine," causes many men to funnel all their emotions into sex or aggression (the third commandment), and this in turn causes affection to always be associated with sex (the fourth commandment). If these commandments stay in place, they can keep a man imprisoned within a dysfunctional structure.

But imagine some big game of Jenga, or pulling a bottom support from a house of cards, and how that affects the whole structure. The same can be done when a man begins to question, or better yet, *replace* the command-ments in his life with healthier beliefs. This may cause the outdated struc-ture to collapse, freeing him up to examine his life and begin living on his own terms. While in theory that may seem like an easy enough task, some men may really struggle with letting go of even one of these command-ments. It takes a lot of determination and hard work; after all, these are "truths" that have been ingrained in most men in their formative years, which means they are particularly hard to shake. Adding to the difficulty is that many of the commandments have a painful emotional legacy attached to them. To work through these commandments means revisiting raw past events that helped create them. You, as a partner, parent, or friend, can learn to be there for the man in your life as he struggles through each one.

## WAKE-UP CALL:
### Commandment Conflict

Take a moment and consider the man in your life; go down the list of commandments and check each one that seems to apply to his particular struggles. You may even write down a specific example that illustrates the conflict to determine the command-ment's intensity. Both the number of commandment conflicts and their intensity will give you a rough estimate of the impact they have on him. This in turn will also give you an idea of how much work may lay ahead for him. Conflicts that are long-term can have a draining effect, not only on his notion of being a man but also on his ability to give extra energy to other areas like work, love, and connecting with you. Think about how we all have a limited amount of psychological energy. If he burns a good por-tion of it trying to keep old conflicts and struggles at bay, it will eventually have an impact across the board. After all, he runs into his notion of being a man in every single aspect of his life from employee/employer, to husband, father, and friend.

# CHAPTER CUES

1. While "The Ten Commandments of Growing Up Male" seem set in stone, they are actually rules that society has made up over the past 100 years or so.

2. Many of the commandments are interlocked and interrelated.

3. The commandments are often confusing and contradictory in nature, asking men to be someone they are not.

4. The commandments ultimately restrict a man's potential in the areas of work and love; they keep him from becoming his own man.

5. No man can keep all the commandments.

6. Men can rewrite the commandments to fit who they really are.

# 2

# The Secret Shoe Box:
# The Basis for Love and Sex

nderstanding how men are socialized to view their emotions and
bodies, and the resulting conflicts that emerge from this view, is an
important step in unlocking the secret lives of men. Interwoven
into each of the next three chapters is a key concept we will refer to as
"emotional compression." This refers to the side effect(s) that occur when
conflicted emotions are not dealt with directly.

Let's start with the fundamental premise that significant conflict does not
magically disappear from the psyches or hearts of human beings, but
instead seeks to be discharged, expressed, and resolved. If a conflict is
intense enough, and no direct path is available, then indirect avenues may
be used. When the psychological pressure cooker of emotional compression blows, it can result in behavior such as slips of the tongue in otherwise
polite conversation, evocative dreams that leave the dreamer startled, emotions that appear in masked form, and even in disturbing troubles that are
funneled into physical symptoms within the body.

Another important aspect about emotional compression is that the
harder a person works at distancing himself from conflicted emotional
material, the greater the chances are he will become confused or disconnected from what is really going on in his internal world. After all, it is very

hard to say, "I will only allow myself to feel certain kinds of emotions" without running the risk of either losing touch with or distorting other feelings and bodily sensations. The end result is the inability to develop a sense of mastery over what is sensed and felt. This is a real problem that can lead to common misunderstandings, like tender feelings being confused with sexual feelings by those who mistake emotional intimacy for physical intimacy (to name just one example).

Further, the compression effect is intensified when there are only a few socially sanctioned methods of expressing a wide repertoire of emotional experiences. Those in the field of men's psychology have noted that male socialization seems to encourage men to funnel all vulnerable feelings into sex or aggression, whether they actually belong there or not. While some avenues close, others, such as the body, a symbol of strength and prowess, are opened. The body can be used to hide masculine insecurity or simply to shield others from seeing human emotions that are considered off-limits. This may include doing a "man-up" by hitting the gym a little too hard, a little too often, but also by training oneself to never let anyone see you sweat in other ways (e.g., emotionally).

But what happens when men begin to lose the body as a shield? While antiaging products seem to stereotypically belong on the other side of the gender aisle, men do not always gracefully accept that their corporeal being has a limited number of miles, no matter how much Viagra, plastic surgery, or steroids beg to differ. It is not just vanity that compels men to use these products, but rather a desperate attempt to keep the body afloat in order to retain a viable sense of masculinity.

Taken together, these various areas have the potential to be confusing and to cause trouble not only for a man but also for those he loves. After all, one of the most common complaints about a man is that he doesn't talk about emotions. Given the liabilities involved in male socialization, the real problem with not being able to show emotion may actually involve some combination of not feeling safe enough to reveal that part of himself, or that he actually does not know how.

In this chapter, we will focus on the emotional basis for intimacy and, in turn, sex. Many of the stereotypical complaints within a long-term relationship involve the sexual aspects: "Our sex life is not what it used to be," or "We never seem to be in sync about having sex; either one person can't get enough or the other acts as though it's a household chore." We will draw from Chapter 1's focus, highlighting how some of the Ten Commandments of Growing Up Male in contemporary society affect love and sex. Some of the struggles resulting from these commandments make men susceptible to confusion in matters of the heart and a little bit further south in their anatomy as well.

Regarding emotions, men perceive a need to put shields up in order to keep prying eyes from seeing their innermost worlds. In their training to become men, boys quickly learn not to leave themselves open to too much vulnerability because it might result in distressing consequences in the social sandbox of males, a hierarchy based on strength and power. But this is not always a gender-exclusive bias; girls and women also know the well-worn blueprint for accepted maleness. Both genders can be quick to point out when perceived commandment breakers make themselves known.

Keeping up perceptions can have an impact on both the inner and outer worlds of boys; eventually problems can develop and follow them into adulthood. All parties are lulled into believing that men's semblance of being sufficient islands unto themselves is a healthy reality, but actually, this prescribed behavior often masks a deeper sense of isolation. A void is created that can only be filled by another person(s) who makes it safe to temporarily set aside the persona of abject self-reliance and reveal what lies in a deeper place. This can include a desire for tenderness, or the sharing of disturbing unresolved conflicts from the past; still other times, there is a terrible longing to be understood, accepted, and even appreciated for the genuine person beyond the male guise, which has been years in the making.

When I told friends I was writing about the secret lives of men, I got some interesting reactions. The most straightforward comment was "You're going to get your ass kicked!" The funny thing is, it was only women who told me that revealing the inner world of males would bring such a terrible uproar from men. One of the more compelling comments that sparked this book was when a friend of mine half-jokingly said that his marriage would be much improved if he had a manual that his wife could consult to learn about his needs. While such a guide might include certain stereotypical aspects associated with maleness, like her willingness to accept gift certificates from lingerie stores or a signed release for an occasional night out with the boys, what he wanted her most to understand was what it is like for him when he is in a tough place emotionally and what she could do to be supportive. Even more important, he wanted her to understand how crucial it is that she appreciate and value him for who he really is, not the version he often feels pressured into being by others.

Bruce Springsteen's ballad "Secret Garden" speaks of a metaphoric place inside of a woman. It is the deepest, most genuine part of her, hidden from the world, and only the luckiest can gain access to it. Is there a male equivalent to a woman's secret garden? I think so. Creating a new metaphor for our purposes here, let's call it "the secret shoe box." Now at first glance, a secret garden and a secret shoe box seem vastly different, but one of the most important secrets revealed in this book is that in the realm of psychological and emotional needs, men and women are far more alike than different. This includes the desire to be valued for who you genuinely are, the wish to receive support in times of need, and the necessity to develop an internal strength that enables you to stand behind personal convictions, protecting yourself and those you love. These are not gender-specific needs and desires; they are human ones. The secret shoe box, just like the secret garden, has the capacity to become a holding place of meaning and creativity.

# The Secret Shoe Box

Imagine you were lucky enough to find a collection of what a preteen boy holds dear. You might find a shoe box hidden in the bottom of a closet, under his bed, or under a loose floorboard. In this box, you might find a picture of his idol on a baseball card or the statistics of his favorite sports team clipped from the newspaper. You may find something that his father gave him that signifies a special shared moment. Of course, you would see a picture of his first crush, a cheerleader at school or a movie star dressed in a bikini. But there are a load of intangibles also placed in this secret shoe box: worries about measuring up as a man, doubts from the multiple competitions that he has endured, confusion about sexual feelings, and, of course, the pure joy, playfulness, curiosity, and wonder that springs from the eternal joy of being a boy.

The contents in this shoe box are precious and represent what a boy holds dear to his heart. This box is his "holy of holies," but he learns there is good reason to keep it hidden from sight. These treasures represent the budding notion of his private self—that part of him that is composed of his most personal memories, thoughts, and feelings. This is healthy and good; he is valuing himself by being careful regarding with whom he shares this treasure. Another, less healthy reason to keep these things to himself is connected to the rules he learned about being a man. The commandments won't allow the outward display of some behaviors. What is contained within this shoe box could cause him trouble if it falls into the wrong hands; the contents could be used against him at the most inopportune time. Often there are discernible events punctuating the extreme vulnerability associated with the materials in his box; he learns after a certain age that it is time to block almost everyone from access to this magical container. He swears the secret shoe box is locked away for good, but as he grows into an adult, he sometimes comes back to it, depositing special moments that affect his life. Sometimes these are good experiences, like falling in love, achieving success in his job, or having his best friend watch his back in the most difficult of circumstances.

All the contents of the secret shoe box are genuine and authentic. However, this doesn't mean these items only represent the warm experiences that make a man endearing to a woman. Things that are real and true can be authentically disturbing and difficult to bear as well. Sometimes these experiences are heartbreaking, filled with anger and remorse: misunderstandings from the formative years that were so intense they left a mark, aspects from adulthood like ugly divorces or custody fights for kids. Sometimes, when the box is opened and shared with another, the first whiff of its contents may be putrid, biting, or stale. Men know this on some level, and that fact gives them all the more reason to keep the lid closed and the contents hidden.

What is perplexing about this secret shoe box is that as much as a man fears letting someone else see the contents, he would truly like to feel safe enough to reveal it and tell the story of each item. After all, they represent a man's innermost self. This is especially true with the people most dear to him. Sometimes he has been waiting a good part of his life for all the contents to be known by another. He may take out one item for show-and-tell only to find out his loved one does not understand its meaning. If this goes badly, the item goes back in, and extra precautions are taken so that the shoe box will not be shared again.

Each man, whether friend, family member, or romantic partner, has this collection that contains the good, the bad, and the ugly. He would like to feel safe enough with you to open the box in your presence and show you what is inside, yet simultaneously he fears that you will fail him; after all, experience has taught him that many people will not "get" him, and they may actually use this material against him. Later we will see how you can help make the man in your life feel safe enough to open up this secret shoe box.

It is probably already clear to you how this fits into our discussion on love and sex. The shoe box is the foundation upon which the deepest emotional connections are built. For a romantic relationship, this will be a core aspect of satisfying sex. While some men may report that sex is just sex, a physical release with no real emotional meaning, a man who has truly made love to a woman opens up the secret shoe box and shares a part of himself. Whether a passionate encounter or a tender one, the most meaningful and "hot" sex involves a shared intimacy with another person. The man in your life wants to feel free enough to share who he is with you. He wants you to be his confidant and lover.

**RELATIONSHIP RED ZONE:**
**Recognizing Secret Shoe Box Material**

The ability to recognize secret shoe box material is very important. Usually there will be certain telltale signs that your man has opened the box and is revealing an important aspect in his life. He might give you an obvious turn signal in the conversation, announcing what a big deal it is for him. He may say something like, "I have never told anyone this before," or "When I have told this to other people in the past, they have not understood," or, "This is hard for me to talk about." All of these and comments like them announce the impending disclosure of important information.

Another very reliable gauge is the sudden appearance of emotion as he talks. In the next chapter on man emotions, you'll learn more about the subtle nuances in these appearances, but for now, realize that when he speaks about something close to the heart, emotions are not far from the surface. These emotions can include regret, sadness, joy, pride, anger—you name it. Once you understand the varying degrees in how men express emotions outwardly, you'll be able to recognize the blip on the radar screen that shows you when emotionally energized talk is different than normal.

# The Confusion Between Libido and Sex

A potential stumbling block for many men is knowing the difference between libido and sex. To explain this confusion, we will have to address a widely misrepresented notion, one that even finds its way into many psychology 101 university courses. It usually occurs when students are introduced to Freud. I know, I know—people have immediate reactions to him, like "that old perv." Freud is a difficult read for a number of reasons; his theories evolved over time, and he was not always clear about the revisions. At the time, people did not have those daily computer downloads updating the new psychoanalytic software. Also, sometimes finding English words to convey the exact meaning or complexity in German is challenging, so ideas can get lost in translation.

One of the key examples of this was Freud's notion of "libido," often mistakenly taught as referring to only the lascivious aspects of sex. Let's be clear: Freud created "drive theory," which emphasizes a psychological need to express and thereby reduce certain physical/psychological tensions back to homeostasis or balance, and he did talk about sex as one of the drives that needed release. However, with libido, this concept is actually more complicated than most people give him credit for; Freud was actually trying to explain the basis for all human connection. He called this "libido," which is derived from the German *liben*, translated as "to love." Libido refers to, as Freud tells us, the "tender feelings" shared between two people. Relationships involving libido can include nonsexual relationships such as mother/son, father/daughter, and male and female best friends, as well as relationships of a romantic nature. The common link is the tender feelings that are invested in one another. While others in psychoanalysis took this emphasis much further, stating that the quintessential human drive was not sex and aggression but rather the need for connection itself, Freud's notion of libido is important to understand.

Sometimes I ask parents in my psychology classes, "Are you in love with your children?" Some will react with shock to this because they automatically associate "being in love" with wanting to have sex. When I explain to them that the investment of libido in someone is the same as investing love energy in them, the confusion goes away. The same is true when Valentine's Day rolls around and you ask someone to be your valentine;

what you are essentially doing is asking, "Can I invest my libido/love energy in you?" Imagine on the next February 14 all the little kids in America going from desk to desk in their classrooms, giving their classmates cards and candy with the "Be my valentine" message. Are we starting them early in the art of seduction by teaching them skills to be used later during some pickup scenario in a bar? No! We are teaching them about libido and the various ways it can manifest itself: sometimes in friendship with same-sex peers, sometimes with an opposite-sex friend, and sometimes as a budding romantic crush. All of these are based on love energy, or libido.

Libido is the basis for all relationships that involve tender feelings. Sex, however, is associated with a special type of relationship that is romantic in nature. Not everyone you have a libidinal or love-energy investment in is also a candidate for a passionate or sexual encounter. This can confuse a lot of people, especially men. In men's training, they are usually not taught the difference between libido and sex; often they learn that they are the same thing. This confusion is the basis for many homophobic reactions in men, because they are taught that feeling emotionally connected to someone always implies wanting to have sex with that person. I try to counteract this reaction in men by drawing on one of my favorite examples of libidinal investment among men.

Larry McMurtry's Pulitzer Prize–winning novel *Lonesome Dove*, later turned into an Emmy-winning miniseries, tells the story of two old, crusty Texas Rangers in the late nineteenth century. In the miniseries, the Rangers are played brilliantly by Robert Duvall and Tommy Lee Jones. After spending most of their adult lives together taming the Wild West in Texas, the semiretired Rangers decide they want to be the first to raise cattle in Montana, so they drive a herd of longhorn cattle from south Texas to Montana.

The cattle drive is a typical plot element in lots of Westerns, but what is not typical is how McMurtry portrays the relationship between the two Texas Rangers. Their relationship includes a good bit of the expected banter, but what comes through in certain moments is the true essence of their friendship and connection. These old guys have spent a lifetime watching each other's backs, seeing each other's failed relationships with women, and drinking too much in each other's company. Toward the end of the story, one of the Rangers falls prey to an Indian's arrow and is on his deathbed while the other one tends to him. You can stack the moving quality of this death scene shared between two friends alongside any in literature. I remind both men and women of the serious libidinal investment between these tough old Texas Rangers.

## Can Men and Women Really Be Friends?

In the now-classic movie *When Harry Met Sally*, Billy Crystal suggests to Meg Ryan on their first of many meetings that men and women can never truly be friends because the "sex thing always gets in the way." This theme in the movie has no doubt led to a number of dinner party debates about the possibility of platonic friendship between the sexes. The movie ultimately concludes not only that men and women can be friends, but in the best cases, their friendship is the basis for a lasting, long-term romantic relationship.

But part of the struggle is sorting out when a sense of connection between two people is valued for friendship's sake versus turning into something more than just being friends. *When Harry Met Sally* drives home our previous topic of libido versus sex. Men are taught that emotional intimacy always equals physical intimacy. Men save the secret shoe box for a very select few, which means, in most cases, a potential romantic partner. It is part of the stereotypical wooing process when he risks sharing more of himself for the woman he loves. This is seen as a heroic feat. So when a man opens up the secret shoe box to a woman, he is trained to believe this is always the next step in romantic foreplay. Unfortunately, this is not always the case and sometimes leads to relationship complications with friends or other would-be emotional supports.

I remember when I really learned the difference between libido and sex.

I was twenty-five years old and in graduate school, training to be a psychologist. During this time, I was introduced to my own personal therapist, who bore a striking resemblance to Dr. Ruth Westheimer, the noted sex therapist. After talking with her for a number of months about all matter of personal things within my own secret shoe box, including my family and current girlfriend, one night I had a startling dream. In the dream, there was a woman, who I quickly identified as my current girlfriend, standing before me dressed in rather sexy lingerie. But what happened next was quite a surprise. My vision in the dream panned like a camera up from the floor, starting with my girlfriend's feet, then legs, then torso, and finally up to her head. To my shock, this woman had the body of my girlfriend but the head of my therapist! The dream-camera pulled back to a full-length shot, and there stood a woman who was the combination of the two women I was currently "involved with." I woke up from the dream with a start and instantly thought about canceling my next appointment with my therapist. After a cold shower, I began to settle down, but I still had worries about bringing this up in my next therapy appointment.

The next week I rather sheepishly approached the topic, wondering if I would be kicked out of therapy for the libidinal Frankenstein creature I had created in my dream. To my shock and amazement, my Dr. Ruth look-alike calmly explained to me that I was learning a valuable lesson about intimacy. "Some people you care about," she said, "you learn to place in one type of intimacy box, and others in another." It seemed very simple after that explanation; there were different types of intimacy—emotional and physical—and they were not always combined in every type of caring relationship. And that was that. I never had anymore dreams about my therapist, because she had been sorted out and placed in the box that was associated with a different kind of intimacy that had nothing to do with sex, but everything to do with libido.

> ### WAKE-UP CALL:
> ### Areas Where Libido and Sex Can Get Confused
>
> For some men, the confusion between libido and sex can be found in a number of different relationships:
>
> - Professional, helping relationships with a therapist or doctor
> - Relationships with close female friends
> - Relationships that have a mothering quality to them
> - In some cases, libido can take a twisted turn. This can involve children and stepchildren who are placed into the role of emotional confidant and partner. Children are suddenly promoted to adult status and asked to be the parent's best friend. Needless to say, clearing up this confusion sometimes requires professional help.

# The Mind Is the Most Powerful Sex Organ

One may arguably conclude that human beings are driven toward connection with others and that one way it manifests itself is in sexual ways. Commercials for perfumes and colognes get a lot of mileage from overplaying the influence of hormonal sexuality, seemingly leading the charge on what we find arousing, but the truth is that the direction of our innate sexual feelings is ultimately controlled in our hearts and minds. In the first part of this chapter, we saw how libido is the basis for all our tender-feeling relationships, including those that may turn into romantic ones.

The examination of some of the psychological qualities from our most important relationships can reveal what we will eventually find sexually arousing. While we give a nod to biology, it is important to realize that the mind is the most influential sexual organ. This fact is true for both women and men. What people find sexually arousing is based in their own history of emotional desires, wants, and fantasies. Sometimes they desire what they have found emotionally satisfying, while other times they desire what they never had but always wanted. As you may guess, this is a very personal, idiosyncratic process. What excites one individual carries no guarantee of the same effect on that individual's partner. All these aspects are filtered through our psyches and then affect our hearts and sex organs.

What you know about a man's history of being a man will tell you something about what he finds sexually arousing. Some of the basics about how a man is trained by society to be a man will provide the background for this section. As we have discussed, growing up male is not always easy. While some advances have been made, boy culture is still based on a hierarchy of power and strength, governed by often-stringent rules for boys becoming men. We noted how, in the man-making process, boys feel pressured to disassociate themselves from anything that is considered to belong to the world of girls. Unfortunately, through this process they also learn that some normal aspects of being human are off-limits because those aspects are labeled as feminine. These aspects include such qualities as vulnerability, tenderness, and even compromise. The degree to which boys are indoctrinated with these messages will have an influence on what they find sexually arousing.

For instance, a boy who experiences a great deal of harsh training regarding man-making may feel that he can only really enact his manhood by acting out this stringent role with his sexual partner. Occasions when he feels like he is fulfilling this prescription of being a man will be exciting to him. He is essentially following the script he has been taught. He might feel compelled to be a take-charge guy who does not let tenderness or vulnerability ever play any part in his lovemaking. In the very back of his mind, there is a voice whispering to him, applauding him in his efforts as a lover. This is the voice of the person who taught him to be a man.

The thing to consider is this: is any given moment arousing because it feels genuine and consistent with who he is as a man or just with the persona he has been taught to assume? Here we are on slippery ground, because some messages about being "a real man" can be fraught with destructive elements. For example, one client that I worked with imagined that during sex his penis was an "automatic jackhammer." It became a weapon with which to punish women, not to connect with them. His notion of being a man was filled with some skewed messages that had a subsequent influence on what he found sexually arousing. His mother was a chronic alcoholic and drug user who had abandoned him. He had learned that being a man was about "punishing the bitches before they have a chance to get you."

In this situation, some of the wires about being a man—hurt/abandonment and sexual arousal—were crossed. I could understand who he was trying to settle a score with as he punished the women who entered his bed. He might not have liked it, but the image of his mother was sitting there right beside him, still affecting his every action. So we can see that sometimes men's sexual arousal is based in fulfilling scripts of manhood in unhealthy forms. In these cases, sexual arousal is prompted by things that are broken inside, desires to please those who could not be pleased, or making up for those who hurt us. Needless to say, making the settling of scores the basis for what is sexually arousing will not lead to a lasting or satisfying sexual relationship.

I must point out that although the basis for sexual arousal may have its foundation in a person's past, it is not necessarily composed of all broken and destructive elements. It can include experiences that are connected with the people in our lives or families who made us feel special and cared about. It might involve those who even confirmed our genuine and healthy notion of being men. These elements can become the foundation for healthy choices about whom we select as potential love interests and that govern our sexual desires.

It may not be easy for some men to explain in great detail these important experiences or the deep feelings that go with them; they may just know that when they are with the right person, it feels familiar, comfortable, or exciting in a "homey" sort of way. Instead of articulating the emotional checklist men have for a potential partner, it may be easier to associate the needed emotional characteristics with physical attributes. This can form a romantic shorthand for the "must-haves" of a potential partner. Some men may say they prefer blondes, redheads, tall women, or petite women simply because they associate those physical types with excitement or caring, or whatever else is emotionally important to them. They may reduce more intangible wishes to symbolic form where physical characteristics represent the emotional ones they desire.

In addition, some libidinal confusion in adults is about reawakening emotionally frozen parts in the heart and psyche. From the standpoint of a therapist, when a client begins to feel strangely drawn toward me, in an almost childlike-crush way, it is usually based on the resurgence of arrested tender feelings rather than mature sexuality. If the client is asked, "What is it about our connecting that draws you to me?" I can almost guarantee that the attraction is not based in anything physical. Rather, our connection makes the client feel safe or valued, something that has been missing or never experienced in a relationship with another person before. The value in this is that clients can quickly tune in to the qualities they want and need in a potential partner through this process. This new understanding, gained in therapy, will serve as the basis for other, more mature feelings of sexuality that eventually emerge outside the consultation room.

The bottom line in these stories is that, while we usually don't think about it this way, our histories of tender feelings serve as the foundation for the development of our sexual feelings and the things we find arousing. We can initially associate these emotional aspects with the physical character-istics of another person because they are easy to identify and label. However, a more in-depth analysis of the origins of attraction would even-tually uncover some emotional component as the basis. As a woman, you may be curious about what your husband or boyfriend finds sexually attrac-tive about you and what emotional aspect it is tied to. You may save that conversation for a long car ride in the country, but you can bank on the equation that emotional history influences good sex being true for him, whether he realizes it or not.

What is most important is that you know what those key underlying emotional aspects are for you and your partner. While you may recognize their symbolic form in tangible representations like hair color, build, a way of being in the bedroom, and so on, a deeper understanding can help you verbalize the essence of these aspects. In this way, partners can share not only what sexually arouses them, but the deeper emotional foundation upon which that is built.

## ▶ Toolbox Tip: The Foundation for Sexual Feelings

To put the "safe emotion is the foundation for good sex" formula to test, sit down and make a list of the top three romantic relationships you have had. Think about each one of these and try to identify the unique qualities each partner had that impacted the way you felt. For instance, some may have helped you feel safe because they were dependable and reliable; you knew you could call on them when needed and they would be there. Others may have been smart or challenging, making you stretch yourself personally and intellectually. Another may have been fun and exciting, and you remember how much you laughed.

When you can pinpoint the specifics of each relationship, think about how each had an impact on your sexual feelings. Did some of these emotional qualities make you sexually smolder while others caused you to slowly simmer? Doing this exercise will help you identify the emotional foundation you need to open yourself to really good sex. It may also help you realize what you need more of emotionally in your current relationship so that you *can* do this. While the essence of this is important information to share with your partner, you should be careful about saying things like "Yes, I had really smoking sex with my ex-boyfriend because emotionally he was like . . ." Instead, talk to your partner about what you need to open up to him because you love him and want more out of this part of your relationship.

| Name | Emotional Quality | Impact on Sex |
| --- | --- | --- |
| 1. | | |
| 2. | | |
| 3. | | |

# What Is Healthy Anyway?

Questions that may come to mind at this point might include: "Are there some sexual fantasies that are off-limits?" "Does it mean a man is a caveman with skewed masculinity because he likes being rough during sex sometimes?" "Does it mean a man is a pervert because he likes to experiment with new things in his sex life?" One way to funnel all these questions into one is to ask, "Is there one way we should all be aroused and act in sexual encounters?" The short answer is no. All people have their own unique histories that shape what they find arousing. The rule of thumb to bear in mind is that what you choose to respond to sexually is okay as long as it does not harm you or someone else.

The basic minimum for healthy sex is to do no harm to yourself or others. As we mentioned in the section above, sometimes what people find arousing is based in a legacy of hurt, neglect, or brokenness. Beyond the bare minimum rule, there is still a lot of room for potential growth in your sexual relationship; for some this can literally lead to sexual healing by having corrective emotional experiences that counter previous harmful ones. These experiences are based on positive emotional occurrences that allow for movement toward your best self. It is important to discern which aspects (e.g., scratching old wounds or helping you move toward your higher self) are present in your relationships and to what degree.

In some cases, it may feel like a complicated mix. On one hand, you might feel valued and supported by your partner reaching toward sexual growth and fulfillment, while at other times, he does not respond in ways that are needed because of an emotional wound from the past. Knowing the foundations upon which someone bases sexual arousal (and likewise withdrawal) may lead to sorting out issues in order to find lasting sexual fulfillment.

For instance, the love-'em-and-leave-'em Casanova who enjoys the conquest of seduction but not the lasting connection of a relationship does harm to himself and others. He alienates himself from his own chances to be truly happy while also misleading another person. There is no future in this for him if he continues to make this attitude the basis for what he finds sexually arousing. He will soon find himself old and alone.

A man in his midfifties once told me about his long list of sexual conquests; at the time they numbered over five hundred. He would tell me stories about how he seduced a woman only to lose interest when the next one came along. He would receive angry e-mails, phone messages, and the like from jilted women who did not realize that he was actually in pursuit of an older conquest: parental love and acceptance from a mother who was not able to give it. When someone began showing real interest, she was quickly dismissed as not having the right stuff. Only those women who were withholding and hard to pursue sustained his attention.

# The Fear of Women

As mentioned in Chapter 1, as a result of the commandments in the man-making process, men learn early on to distance themselves from the feminine. This includes stereotypical characteristics associated with females like showing emotions, being nurturing, wanting to connect with someone, or showing a more vulnerable side. One of the important points to keep in mind is that many of these characteristics associated exclusively with the "world of women" are in fact universal characteristics for both sexes, even if they are not always acknowledged or condoned. Men want to possess these aspects, but society has told them the qualities are off-limits if they want to be proper men.

Men spend most of their training learning to distance themselves from the very aspects that women have come to symbolize, not realizing they are giving away their own human birthright in the process. They learn to dispose of some of the characteristics they might possess and actually use to the betterment of themselves and others. This abandonment leaves many men at a disadvantage, including, as you might guess, in matters of the heart. This deficiency in turn affects matters of sexuality and arousal.

One of the effects of the man-making process is that some males learn to actually fear women and the characteristics they have come to represent. They are taught that the virtues of being a woman are actually powerful, corrupting forces against being male. Men can have a number of potential reactions when they see woman in all her feminine glory; they can be threatened, afraid, or feel drawn to her because she represents psychological aspects he can never own himself, at least according to society's standards. Since so much of the feminine world is off-limits to stereotypically traditional men, men who aspire to "manliness" come to see "feminine" aspects like the world of emotions as scary, uncharted territory that must not be breached. When they think of women as being capable of controlling and harnessing such powerful and potentially destructive talents, it leaves an impression.

Men may feel unsure about coming into close contact with what may feel like the combustible material of the feminine realm. When the love of a man's life asks him to be more open and to share his feelings, she is asking him to go against the very grain of what he has been taught about being a man. She is inviting him into "her realm," that of the feminine. It is hard to appreciate the difficulty of this from a man's perspective, after he has spent so many years training himself to gain distance from all things feminine. It can feel simultaneously exciting and frightening to be in prolonged contact with any characteristics, people, places—real or symbolic—that represent the feminine.

There is a famous story about Hollywood tough guy Humphrey Bogart. He met nineteen-year-old Lauren Bacall on the set of the movie *To Have and Have Not*. After courtship, they fell in love and eventually married. Bogart, who was nearly twice Bacall's age and a founding member of the notorious Rat Pack, confided to a friend his feelings on his upcoming nuptials. He said he felt like a mouse and his-soon-to-be wife was a lion about to pounce on him.

The fear of women is not a modern concept. Some scholars believe that in prehistoric times, before conception was fully understood, women were considered supernatural creatures. Having yet to connect the act of sex to having babies only amplified men's fears about women, because it seemed as if their bodies could do magical things. Women could produce milk from their breasts, babies from their bodies, and bleed once a month in line with the lunar cycle. In some cultures, women gathered at the time of the planting of crops to sit in the fields where seeds would be placed in order to ensure fertility, because they had the magical powers to bring about the growth of all living things.

Adding to this theme, and consistent throughout Western culture, are myths, legends, and fairy tales about the power of a woman's sex organs. In some of these stories monsters, snakes, or even vicious teeth lived inside a woman's vagina. In many of these stories, the male hero was to have sex with such a woman but also avoid the dangers that inhabited the netherworld of her body. So from a man's perspective, the potential fear of women may stifle matters of the heart as well as affect his arousal. When he becomes involved in a long-term relationship or gets married, a period of adjustment may be needed for him to trust that the woman he loves is safe and won't use her magical powers against him.

Finally, there is another, more positive outcome for men and their struggle with the fear of the feminine. Analyst Carl Jung noted that for men to make peace with this realm, they need to embrace their own feminine characteristics. Statements such as these have often been misinterpreted, subsequently becoming fodder for bad jokes about men being in touch with their "feminine sides." These feminine qualities can be thought of as relational ones, placing an emphasis on connecting with self and others. This means a man learns about being in relationship with himself, being in touch with emotions, bodily sensations, thoughts, and feelings, as well as being capable of forming relationships with other human beings. What society labels as feminine does not always exclusively belong to the world of women. These are skills that both men and women have and can improve. When these relational skills are owned and incorporated, a man can appreciate—instead of fear—the feminine.

## Here Comes a Baby in the Baby Carriage

Sometimes women and men report changes in their sexual feelings after they have a child together. For a woman this may have to do with fluctuating hormones, or with the sheer physical overload of tending to a newborn and feeling too exhausted for sex. The last thing women may want after having a newborn crawl all over their bodies is to have their man tag into the ring and be physical as well. Certainly there can be a psychological adjustment as well to assuming the role of partner, lover, and now, caretaker. Women report the difficulty in adjusting roles, moving from the nursery into the bedroom in one fell swoop, going from breast-feeding to making love.

There can also be a big psychological adjustment for men. Some men will report they just don't feel sexual toward the woman who is now the mother of their child. But why? There can be a couple of reasons that are based on perceived changes of the identity of the woman they love. One of these reasons is summed up in an old psychoanalytic phrase: "Madonna-whore complex." This particular complex represents the dilemma of simultaneously seeing the woman they love and in whom they have invested sexual feelings also transform into a new creature, in this case, a mother. While this may not seem like a tall order, the commandments make this a difficult task. Seeing the object of their sexual desires also becoming maternal is a psychological transition. For some men it feels like their partner has turned into a "new woman." The maternal aspect men are most familiar with is associated with their mothers. The "icky" feeling some men report is that being with this "new mom" feels a little like incest.

The problem is related to the expanding, new identity of their woman — that she can simultaneously be a source of tenderness, sexuality, and maternal virtue. Men may have questions about how to act around her. Are certain things that were okay before off-limits now because she is a mom? Can there still be hot sex? After all, is that the way you treat a mother? When men become fathers, they are also in the process of expanding their own identity, moving further into the adult world of complex roles and responsibilities. If they have received the standard commandment socialization, they may be ill prepared to deal with the added emotional complexity.

In the movie *Nine Months*, Hugh Grant plays a commitment-shy man who finds out his girlfriend is pregnant. While he loves her very much, the thought of being a parent, and even worse, his girlfriend becoming a mother, literally terrifies him. He unconsciously sabotages the relationship at every turn, missing sonogram appointments and being unable to get excited about the pregnancy because of his own fears. He even has a nightmare about his pregnant girlfriend: while they're in bed, she reaches out to him in what he feels is an amorous invitation, but when he rolls over he finds that his beautiful girlfriend has been transformed into a praying mantis — the female known to eat the male after they mate.

I have heard a number of stories about the actual birthing process affecting men's sex drive. A woman once told me that her husband fainted in the delivery room as her cervix dilated to birthing size. I can just imagine what was going through his mind: "My God, I have married an alien creature. If you think I am ever going back down there again, you're crazy!" The long-story-short is that for some men it will take time to adjust to being with this "new woman."

If they have not already done so, men are forced to confront the sometimes confusing world of libido and sex when they become involved in a committed relationship — and then when children come along, men have to work through yet another level of the complicated nature of love. They have to understand that a woman can simultaneously be the source of sexual and maternal feelings, and they must also come to grips with the new magical powers their superhero wife has developed in birthing a child.

What happens when the amorous deck of cards is reshuffled, or in this case when new cards are added, is that some men have to rethink what is going on. They may have questions, fears, or uncertainties (as well as joys) that need to be talked about in order to get back on track. While I have been stressing some of the potential troubles, the fear of the feminine does not affect all men. Some are able to look at pregnant women and conclude with a rush of excitement, as Big Daddy did in Tennessee Williams's play *Cat on a Hot Tin Roof,* "That woman has got life in her!"

# Conclusion

For human beings, sexual arousal is largely governed by the mind. What excites someone sexually is tied to emotional needs and fantasies as much as it is to physical stimulation. Arousal draws upon the individual's unique history of relationships, both healthy and damaging. As we will see in more depth later in the book, the chase for some present-day romantic partners is really based in confronting ghosts from the past. A man may be trying to make up for past emotional wounds with both Mom and Dad. Complicating matters of the heart is the constraining nature of the commandments; they stifle a man's ability to freely share with others, both partners and friends, and keep him from sharing the contents of his shoe box. We will see there are ways to alleviate these situations that involve men employing the secret shoe box as a source of creativity and connection rather than convolution and confusion.

# CHAPTER CUES

1. Men have a secret shoe box where they keep the most personal aspects of themselves.

2. Your partner's ability to feel safe enough to share the contents of the shoe box with you will make for a better sex life. Emotional intimacy is the basis for the most satisfying physical intimacy.

3. Libido, love energy, or tender feelings are the basis for all our caring relationships, including romantic ones.

4. Sometimes libido and sex are confused by both men and women.

5. What we find sexually arousing is based in our unique histories of tender feelings.

6. Sometimes what is experienced as sexually arousing is based on trying to please important people from the past.

7. Sometimes what is experienced as sexually arousing is based on trying to experience unfulfilled emotional needs from the past.

8. Tangible turn-ons like hair color, body type, and attitudes in the bedroom are often symbolic ways to represent the emotional needs that make sex most satisfying.

9. Verbalizing the tangible and deeper emotional aspects to your partner results in a better sex life.

10. The rule of thumb for healthy sex is to do no harm to yourself or others.

11. Marriage and having babies can lead to a fear of the feminine; men need to rethink their own roles and identities, as well as those of their partners.

# 3

# Man Emotions:
# More than Sex and Aggression

In Charles Darwin's famous study, *The Expression of the Emotions of Man and Animals* (1872), he concluded that human beings share a species-wide repertoire of emotional expressions. The universal emotional expressions included fear, surprise, anger, disgust, sadness/grief, and joy/happiness. That is, everyone, men and women alike, experienced and expressed these reactions. He believed that natural selection actually facilitated having everyone on the same level in terms of a basic set of emotions, thereby allowing the human species to communicate more effectively.

In spite of Darwin's theory about emotions, this area causes much of the contention experienced between men and women. Since Darwin's work, the theme of universal hardwired human emotions has evolved as others have echoed similar conclusions. There is contemporary support provided by both biologists and psychologists concerning the existence of basic emotions and their expression, referred to as "primary emotions." There are also "secondary emotions" that are heavily influenced by cultural attitudes and socialization. These feelings are used as substitutes or defenses for primary emotions when the "normal" reactions break cultural taboos or may be too emotionally overwhelming.

To see the power of the secondary emotions in action, let's take a research study comparing Japanese to Americans while watching stressful films. As expected, based on cultural mores that emphasize a taboo on public displays of strong "negative" emotion, especially with strangers, Japanese subjects showed markedly more stoic responses. When asked face to face about the stressful films, they politely smiled, masking what they considered culturally negative feelings. However, the researchers videotaped each of the subjects' facial expressions in these interviews, and the tape revealed that they had, in a fraction of a second, shown the characteristically negative emotional expression and then quickly replaced it by a more culturally acceptable one. Also, when the Japanese subjects watched the films alone, believing no one was observing them, their facial expressions were the same as the Americans. In this study, Japanese subjects had learned to use secondary emotions to mask their primary ones.

It would not be a big leap from the example above to see how the power of gender expectations sometimes governs people's emotional responses. Those emotions considered appropriate for one gender but not for the other may lead to the use of secondary emotions. When this happens, an emotional detour can occur, making things confusing for the person experiencing the emotion(s) and for the person observing them. This can lead to a breakdown in communication as well as people losing touch with what they actually experience.

I would be preaching to the choir if I said that some men have a tenuous relationship with emotions. You may actually know men who see emotion as something to keep in check or gain mastery over, especially if you understand how primary and secondary emotions get mixed up. Due to the commandments, men are taught to have an uneasy relationship with feeling things. They learn early on that doing so can often lead to showing the cards they are playing. Others may pick up on what is hidden and potentially use any exposed, incriminating material against them.

In some ways, men who can master the art of the poker face, even in the midst of intense emotion, have an advantage; it's like building a big wall around the perimeter of your house. People who are curious about the goings-on inside that dwelling never get a clear view. Without the ability to clearly see within people base their perceptions on what they see and only guess about what's blocked from view. Likewise, men's blank expressions act as a barrier, sometimes baffling others into making erroneous conclusions. People may believe there is nothing going on inside of them, or worse, that men don't even have emotions. While every man feels things, he may not always show it, fess up to it, or even recognize it. While a man's emotional life is often cloaked, it doesn't mean there is nothing going on; it's just that men have learned through their man-training to go underground with their feelings or to mask them.

In the last chapter, we learned about the secret shoe box, or the metaphorical place where a man stores his innermost thoughts, feelings, and memories. The commandments allowed few outsiders to have full access to this treasure trove, sometimes including the man himself. Emotional compression occurs with this process of trying to keep the lid on tightly, even as new and sometimes multifaceted items are added to the box. We saw this earlier when considering libido and sexual arousal; there are such subtle differences between these two emotions that they can often be confused when crammed too tightly into the same psychological space or when the proper emotional maturing has not occurred. A man needs to take emotions like these out of the secret shoe box in order to learn, practice, and gain a sense of mastery over them. If they never see the light of day, chances are they will go unrealized and fall short of their full potential.

Another aspect of the compression effect of the secret shoe box is that feelings are expressed through indirect means, in this case, masked by the use of secondary emotions. They may be expressed in less orthodox ways when the normal channels are off-limits. If men cannot express emotions directly, or even allow themselves to acknowledge what is in the secret shoe box, they will still find a route of conveyance. Emotions must go somewhere. Sometimes this occurs in unconscious ways, like dreams, slips of the tongue, or bodily symptoms such as chest pain.

Under the guidance of the commandments, boys are trained not to express socially unauthorized emotions such as pain, vulnerability, and all those things falsely labeled as feminine. Boys learn to mask these emotions. We will see a major example of this in the way vulnerability is cloaked as aggression. The outside observer who is not privy to such things might conclude that the male is just an angry young man. There is no recognition that the genuine emotion—a deep hurt that he can ill afford to fully reveal—has been successfully disguised. As one may imagine, this leads to problems in communication with others, and after so many years of this internal sleight of hand, he even loses touch with himself. He may not really know what he feels because the lines of the true nature of his feelings have been blurred. The cloaking technique has been too effective.

So, in terms of the emotional masking technique, think about a box of crayons with each subtle shade representing an individual emotion or some derivation of it. In the normal part of the human experience, if we were to acknowledge the entire emotional package, we would need one of those 64- or 124-crayon boxes; there are many different things to feel. But, due to their training, men are not allowed to have so many crayons in their box.

In this chapter, we will explore the two areas where men have an outward and acknowledged sense of emotion: sex and aggression. I will warn you ahead of time that these two areas are much more complex than you might think at first glance. Hidden in that seemingly nearly empty box of two crayons are actually lots of subtle shades. Eskimos have multiple definitions and nuances for the single word "snow." They have a word for wet snow, icy snow, snow that is foreboding, and snow that is good for travel. These different gradations of the same word for what seems like the same thing may be puzzling to an outsider. But for Eskimos, multiple uses of the same word are born from necessity. What seems like a simple thing at first glance is actually very complex upon further inspection. I believe that many men's use of the words *sex* and *aggression* is similar to the Eskimos' use of the word *snow*. At first glance, it seems fairly simple, but in reality it is complex and multidimensional.

You will notice that many of the multidimensional uses of sex and aggression as potential primary or secondary emotions do not belong exclusively to the realm of men. Women reading this chapter will recognize themselves as well, because, just like men, they are hardwired for a full range of emotions, including sexual feelings and aggression. Also, those who have grown up in a particular era or have undergone similar cultural or family socialization may make use of the comparable kinds of techniques or repertoire of secondary emotions. The specific use of secondary emotions should be expected to cross the gender line when backgrounds are similar. For instance, a woman who grew up in a family that placed emphasis on the stiff-upper-lip approach to life or a strong emphasis on achievement may adopt some of the attitudes and behaviors stereotypically associated with traditional masculine values, including how emotions are expressed (look no further than Lara Croft movies or a few characters from *Sex and the City*). Some women may ask, "Are you saying I am acting like a man?" No, you're just using some techniques that have been traditionally associated with a "man's world."

As stereotypical gender roles become less stringent, as they have over the past forty years, men and women discover more and more that some things labeled as belonging exclusively to one sex are actually accessible to everyone in the same species—the human species. This realization may prompt the reader to think through their own history of the dos and don'ts associated with emotions; it may also point back to one of the simple truths interlaced throughout this book: men and women are more psychologically alike than different, but stereotypical gender socialization can lead people to conclude they are as different as two planets. So, while this chapter reveals more about the secret lives of men, it will also reveal what men and women have in common.

# Sexual Feelings

Men may have many different types of uses for the word "sex." Some of these versions you may not be aware of, and others you may not want to be connected with, but there can be both positive and negative sides to these aspects. There is a tendency for this topic to be evocative, which is one of the reasons that it becomes a potential difficulty in relationships. It can conjure up insecurities and painful images from the past, and for some it is an area they just don't feel comfortable discussing.

To make our way through these potential obstacles, let's try to place sex in a different perspective. For many people, differing conceptions of sex are related to what life stage a person is in and the level of connection they are seeking with their partners. Also, some of these differing aspects of sex are more in keeping with a particular man's goal, while others subtract from his aims.

The definitions and components of what feels like *appropriate* sex may vary for individuals over the course of their lives. In other words, context has a lot to do with how we view sex. A teenager will look at sex much differently than a senior citizen. Often what feels right sexually and which avenues to pursue are very personal decisions. Sexual experimentation and exploration usually begins in early adolescence and then evolves somewhat during the college years. For many, the college years are a time of separating from the family, exploring the world, and discovering more about "adult" sex and sexuality. Some will take this to the extreme in a "girls or boys gone wild" fashion, while others explore to a lesser degree. The aim in this phase of life is to investigate and set the stage for the possibility of more mature loving relationships. This is accomplished through dating or meeting different types of people. Romantic interest and varying degrees of sexual exploration are a natural part of this.

Sexual goals in different life stages impact the meaning of sex in other ways. For instance, those who are in the early stages of committed relationships and are trying to build a life together may be especially challenged or harmed when there is infidelity. Intimacy issues and conflicts can sometimes masquerade as sexual troubles. A man in his late twenties confided to me that while he loved his wife very much, the thought of being "tied down" to just one woman seemed "suffocating." He was often tempted to have his "stash" on the side to help with that fear. Take note that using the word "stash" does not even recognize the other woman as a person. His stash seemed to be more about intimacy fears related to being with one person than a hormonal need to procreate with lots of women.

Another sexual scenario might include men and women who are in long-term relationships where the connection is solid. There is no question of loving and being committed to each other, but after years of the same positions and routines, they want to put some spice into their romantic life. They may do this through role-playing, games, toys, or whatever works for the couple. Even in the twilight years, notions of sex may still evolve for some. Some may be surprised that recent research suggests a growing risk of sexually transmitted diseases among the postretirement crowd. With the high number of widows and widowers seeking company in various forms, naturally some of this will lead to having sex. For some this may feel like a second adolescence where there is dating but without the previous sexual restraints of youth.

Yet another aspect to consider about differing personal notions of sex is the desired quality of emotional connection between sexual partners. For instance, if the person you are with is basically a faceless other whose main purpose is to reduce sexual tension, you wouldn't expect any real intimacy there. In contrast, there are those people who really are in love and want to make a baby together as an expression of their union. There is no forced choice between these two sexual options—no real intimacy or solely spiritual types of sex. Couples who love each other should enjoy the playful aspects as well. They can explore, try new things, and do what feels consistent to maintain and enhance their solid connection. Likewise, those who have intimacy as one of the items on their to-do list can make strides as well.

Beyond life stages and intimacy levels, a man's personal goals also affect the different versions of sex he may be interested in. Various types of sex can be in keeping with his goals or can subtract from his aims. For instance, some of the definitions discussed in this chapter would not enhance a relationship that has any hope of being long-term, much less help him find his true love. A man who bordered on sexual addiction once told me that the reason he had a nonstop string of sexual flings was that he was in search of true love. I was surprised by his answer and thought that he had chosen a funny way to pursue his goal. Naturally, then, a person's sexual history is often a complex matter. This can include some natural evolution in terms of what feels like appropriate change in sexual behavior across the life span. Many individuals may have tried various forms of sex described in this chapter but grew out of them, realizing they simply do not fit into their lives anymore.

Having established some aspects involved in shaping different definitions of sex and how they are formed and potentially implemented, let's look at the specific types in detail. These include: Man Valium Sex, Hallmark Card Sex, Lustful Sex, Exploratory Sex, Power and Submission Sex, Procreation Sex, Makeup Sex, Checked-out Sex, the Drunken Shag, and Casual Sex. In most cases there are positive and negative aspects for each type. It is stressed throughout that consensual decisions and good communication are necessary skills for a healthy sex life in any relationship.

## Man Valium Sex

In Man Valium Sex, men use sex to sooth themselves from unsettling feelings. There is a physiological as well as psychological release associated with sex and orgasm. In terms of the body, there is a chemical release that actually causes a sedating effect and puts some men to sleep. Some evolutionary scholars believe that this sleepy effect helped a man bond emotionally to the woman by keeping him physically closer longer. It's good to understand that a man is wrestling with his own physiology after sex. Don't take it personally if he is worthless afterward; he is yielding to a biological imperative. In most cases, Man Valium Sex is fine. It can also be the launching pad for other forms of intimacy, like talking about what made it a tough day. Couples just need to work out their pattern for what happens first—sex or talking? However, this type of sex can be problematic if it's the only way a man knows how to soothe troubled or conflicted feelings. Men who come home from a hard day at the office may put the moves on their partner, not understanding that they feel like they are heading to the medicine cabinet for a few aspirins to take the edge off their day.

## Hallmark Card Sex

This is what we normally think of as "making love." A man opens his heart and shares his body with the person he loves in order to feel emotionally close. These are the moments when sex is clearly about deep connection and intimacy. This is the stuff of Hollywood romances and Harlequin novels. Sex is experienced as intense, shared oneness between partners. It may border on a spiritual experience. A challenge may arise if one or both partners feel that each sexual encounter has to be this type. For instance, the stereotype that women have sometimes been sold is that this is the only legitimate brand of sex and all others are illegitimate posers. When an encounter is not a Hallmark Card Sex one, some may react with guilt, feel dirty, or think that their partner or they are "pervs." Men, on the other hand, have been told throughout much of their man-training that this type of sex smacks of all the "feminine" aspects of vulnerability, intimacy, and tenderness that they have been warned against. The fear is that those types of things can corrupt a man's sense of masculinity. Both of these stereotypical messages about sex are fraught with fear and dysfunction — they carry misguided notions.

## Lustful Sex

When a couple has a strong sexual attraction for each other, this may result in a vigorous, lustful type of sex. It may almost seem like there is a chemical reaction going on between the partners, each sending out pheromones, as if their bodies are communicating with each other. This may lead to preoccupation, daydreams and fantasies, or even sexy phone calls and surprise visits. This can include a "nooner" (coming home at lunch for a quickie) because the passion burns. In the cycle of a relation-ship, you might expect this type of experience to be most intense at the beginning, but the embers of the fire can burn throughout the connection.

On the negative side, Lustful Sex gets short-circuited when lust is all there is. A man reported to me that "technically speaking" the best sex he ever had predated his relationship with his wife. He did not feel emotion-ally connected to the women he was with, but felt instead an incredible physical attraction. After the sex was over, there was nothing else. They had no mutual interests, shared values, or any real communication. He said it felt hollow, and they eventually drifted apart because there was nothing to keep them together besides the sex. He said at some point he realized that he wanted a more complete relationship, and soon after that he met his future wife.

## Exploratory Sex

This is the fun, playful type of sex. You might try new positions or intro-duce toys or other arousing stimulation. When couples feel like they are on solid ground emotionally, they are freer to open up to fantasies they have always wanted to explore. In the best situation, this type of sex also has a strong intimacy component, because as you act out a specific fantasy, the part of your psyche that helped create it gets shared as well.

Remember, as we saw in Chapter 2, it is the deeper emotional connec-tions that drive and create our sexual fantasies—the brain is the most pow-erful sexual organ for both men and women. What people find sexually arousing is based on their own unique histories involving emotional needs and desires, and some of this material involves needs that were met while others were unfulfilled. When people act out fantasies, what they are doing is bringing deeper emotional material to life.

Receptive and engaging partners do more than just fulfill playful sex acts in Exploratory Sex; they also give an accepting nod of "you're okay" for having those fantasies and the underlying emotional aspects that helped create them. This accepting approach creates an emotional reaction that may be equally as strong as the actual physical sense of fulfillment. A person shows who he is right down to his own unique variations, including what feels most emotionally and sexually fulfilling.

The potentially problematic aspect of Exploratory Sex can occur when partners are not on the same page in terms of what it is about or where it is headed. Sometimes harsh teaching about sex being dirty and wrong, or that the only legitimate sex is the Hallmark Card type, causes people to approach Exploratory Sex with a cautious eye.

## Power and Submission Sex

For some couples, the use of consensual power and submission can be a form of Exploratory Sex. For them, it is a new way to express and experience their sexual relationship. For others, it can be a regular aspect of an already established way of relating. What is consistent across scenarios, though, is the issue of *power* in the forefront of the sexual encounter. One person has the majority of it, or it is passed back and forth across the encounter(s). For the sake of clarity, this version of sex is defined in terms of the masculine, "aggressive" role in the encounter.

In Power Sex, the man will clearly be the aggressor through becoming very much in touch with his power. In this case, the man calls the shots about what will happen in the sexual encounter. There is the expectation that his partner will go along with his attitude and be receptive to his power. This may include dictating the position(s), use of dirty talk, or rougher sex. There is a clear power differential between partners. Some may react to this negatively, believing that partners should be on equal grounds in terms of power at all times, and that anything less than that is degrading to both parties. But there is an ebb and flow to power in most couples' relationships, and this applies to the area of sex as well.

I remember attending a conference where one of the papers presented was about *Buffy the Vampire Slayer* and how the show was clearly biased against women because all of Buffy's love interests—an assortment of male vampires—"penetrated" her flesh with their fangs. The presenter was especially concerned about the notion of who was penetrating whom, even in this symbolic way. At some point, I could not contain myself any longer and spoke out that when two people really love each other, both people are penetrated—in the heart.

Where this type of sex can go astray is when power expressions are really about giving voice to broken parts in the psyche. Remember the rule from the previous chapter: do no harm to your sexual partner. You may remember from an earlier chapter the example of the man who saw his penis as a punishing jackhammer, wishing to do harm to the women with whom he had sex. This is a prime example of Power Sex going astray.

Submission Sex is when a man's partner is the aggressor. The partner takes the power posture mentioned above and calls the shots. Note that these two different types (Power and Submission Sex) may be reversed throughout a sexual encounter, with one more in control for a time, and then later switching. Couples who share this type of sex move comfortably from power to submissive roles in or across their sexual encounters.

The same cautionary note mentioned above can be restated here. For some, there is a fine line between this type of sex and acting out emotionally damaged parts. Men and women can both feel damaged in the process. A man may enjoy his partner being in control and calling the shots, but the line is crossed when this involves what feels humiliating or degrading. The specific line of what feels appropriate may vary with individual couples. When a foul has been committed, steps can be taken to not only address the situation and make amends but to get on the same page for future encounters, which is all the more reason to have a well-established line of communication regarding the dos and don'ts in your consensual sexual relationship.

## Procreation Sex

This is a special type of sex set aside for baby making. While it can take several forms, the ultimate aim is to get pregnant. It may feel like a lovely ritual where the couple purposefully declares they are ready for the next phase in their connection—having a family. For other couples, this can feel like a different type of sex, especially if there is trouble conceiving. This is due, in part, to the logistics involved in terms of plotting the right fertility time or the most appropriate position for conception. This may include multiple encounters in a short period of time. It may feel more about getting the sperm and egg to successfully meet than engaging in a passionate, intimate encounter.

The potential issues to watch out for in this version of sex have more to do with the meaning attributed to conceiving. Partners may differ in terms of their investment in having a baby, and it may begin to show if conception is difficult or problematic. Partners may experience conflict when these differences become known or even more pronounced when expensive medical bills mount and other logistical sacrifices are made. In addition, it is important to recognize the symbolic significance attached to having a baby. For some, this is a sign that the union is blessed; for others, it means they really are not a family until they have children. When this potentially highly charged, emotional material begins to rise, partners may make accusations or feel like their needs are not being attended to while making concessions for the other person. This cannot only short-circuit sex drives but also undermine the reasons for having the baby.

## Makeup Sex

This is a type of sex that occurs after a fight. We usually don't feel too comfortable with the notion that we can experience competing and conflicting emotions simultaneously, but in Makeup Sex, that's what often happens. One or both partners may feel a blend of emotions during sex. Some partners may feel a thin line between love and anger. Makeup Sex includes the complete emotional package that occurs within a relationship: momentary disdain, hurt, frustration, desire, longing, anger, a desire to reconcile, and intense feelings of love. It can be quite a long list, but it can feel nice to let it all out in a safe way. Makeup Sex is often intensely primal. It loosens the emotional belt and lets everything hang out.

This type of sex can lead to trouble when the best part of the relationship is the making up. Sometimes these sexual encounters can turn into a destructive pattern that includes domestic violence and/or intense emotional abuse. There is a honeymoon phase that follows this type of abuse. It is characterized by the abuser's apologies and promises that things will be different; they may send flowers, be extra sweet, or claim that the relationship really is making a turn for the better now. The victim can feel both relieved there is a respite from the mistreatment and hold to some false sense of hope that things really will be different now because "he promised." This is an "Ike and Tina Turner" type of situation.

## Checked-out Sex

This type of sex occurs in a relationship when a man is not fully in the mood but is a willing participant because his partner wants sex. This may occur in more established relationships or be the product of lots of sex in a brief period of time. Over the course of a relationship, partners may not be in complete sync about sexual urges and intimacies. It happens.

The problematic aspect occurs when being out of sync is the marker for the majority of sexual encounters. In this case, some couples may need to discuss if there are unspoken resentments or other issues that may be blocking a freer interplay of sex. A man told me that he and his wife had very infrequent sexual encounters. She would approach him for sex, and his response was to get his day timer and schedule an appointment during the next week or so for the encounter to occur. He needed to work up to having sex because of unresolved tension that existed in the relationship. While we often think that men are always ready for sex under any conditions, this is quite frankly not true.

In a similar scenario, a man is having sex but he is emotionally checked out or not fully present with his partner. Sometimes this is because of fatigue or intruding thoughts from a long day. Astute partners know when their man feels a million miles away. Often, this is a place to stop sex and say, "What is going on? You don't seem yourself." If handled in a way that deals with the emotionally intruding aspects, what starts out as Checked-out Sex may turn into a more intimate encounter. Talking about troubling things can actually begin to remove potential intimacy barriers.

On the negative side, Checked-out Sex can be a marker for bigger problems. While it is not uncommon for both men and women to have the occasional thought of someone other than their partner during sex, too much of this marks a sign that something is not right. He or she may be fantasizing about someone else because of intimacy problems. There is an episode in *Sex and the City* where one of Miranda's boyfriends must watch porn to be aroused while they have sex; his body is with her but his eyes are on the TV screen. This is a blatant example of a man's penis being engaged while the rest of him is off somewhere else.

## The Drunken Shag

This is a sexual encounter (that may or may not include actual intercourse) where having one too many drinks leads to hookup time. Stereotypically, this can be with a friend, old flame, or a new acquaintance, though it can also occur between seriously committed or married partners of all ages as well. This type of sex is most associated with the exploratory years of college and postcollege and involves intoxicating substances that loosen inhibitions. This type of sex can go astray when the meaning of the encounter is not known or agreed to by both parties. For instance, this may not be the beginning of a relationship, though one party may think so. It can also lead to a greater potential for sexually transmitted diseases (STDs) or pregnancy because of the spontaneity of the moment occurring with a stranger.

## Casual Sex

This is when two parties agree to have a no-strings-attached sexual encounter. There can also be varying versions of Casual Sex, ranging from mere gratification to a tender encounter, to marking "what could have been" if the logistics of life would have permitted the connection to develop. Sometimes people report they wanted Casual Sex because they felt the need for human touch, or because they were lonely, or both.

Casual Sex can occur throughout the life span, but certain versions are more prone in the early adult years. Again, the cautionary tale here is about both partners defining the meaning of Casual Sex; problems arise when either (or both) parties disagree about its significance. Feelings can be hurt, unwanted pregnancies may occur, or STDs can be inadvertently passed between partners.

# Decoding Sex

The importance of knowing these many different shades of sex is this: good sex is ultimately based on communication and consensual decision making. For some couples, a few of these types of sex will not feel right or comfortable. You and your partner will need to discuss and get on the same page about what feels appropriate for the relationship. Objectively speaking, almost all of these types of sex can have a positive spin, but there can be some problematic areas or potential dark sides as well. The next Relationship Red Zone section summarizes both of these possibilities.

## Relationship Red Zone: Secret Decoder Ring for Sex

| TYPES OF SEX | DEFINITIONS |
| --- | --- |
| Man Valium Sex | Used to alleviate unsettling feelings |
| Hallmark Card Sex | Used to emotionally connect with partner |
| Lustful Sex | Pheromones are flying—primal |
| Exploratory Sex | Playful, fun, exploratory in nature |
| Power and Submission Sex | Who is in charge of calling the shots |
| Procreation Sex | Used to conceive a baby |
| Makeup Sex | A gentle blend of anger, love, and reconciliation |
| Checked-out Sex | He is not in the mood but still goes along for the ride. |
| The Drunken Shag | Last call leads to a booty call |
| Casual Sex | Various forms of free love |

| TYPES OF SEX | THE RIGHT WAY |
| --- | --- |
| Man Valium Sex | Can be a soothing release or set the stage for deeper intimacy |
| Hallmark Card Sex | Can be an intense experience that deepens connection |
| Lustful Sex | Intense sexual desire |
| Exploratory Sex | Can lead to playing out fantasies that are accepted by partner |
| Power and Submission Sex | A normal variation in sexual relationship |
| Procreation Sex | Symbolic way of celebrating couple's union |
| Makeup Sex | A way of giving voice to all feelings and making up |
| Checked-out Sex | A willing participant when not really in the mood |
| The Drunken Shag | Can be pleasurable if both parties are on the same page |
| Casual Sex | When both parties knowingly agree to a brief encounter for mutual satisfaction |

| TYPES OF SEX | LEADING TO PROBLEMS |
|---|---|
| Man Valium Sex | When this is the only way he knows how to soothe himself |
| Hallmark Card Sex | When there is an expectation that it should be this way every time |
| Lustful Sex | When lust is all there is |
| Exploratory Sex | When couples are not on the same page about what is acceptable |
| Power and Submission Sex | When broken emotional parts get played on in a damaging way |
| Procreation Sex | May cause stress when there are infertility issues |
| Makeup Sex | When the best part of the relationship is making up |
| Checked-out Sex | When most encounters are of this nature |
| The Drunken Shag | When the meaning of this encounter is not agreed to by both parties |
| Casual Sex | When the meaning of this encounter is not agreed to by both parties |

# Aggression

Well, we've gotten through the sex part, but aggression is another tricky topic because it is equally as evocative as sex for some people. Individual histories can color the notion that any form of aggression is bad and should never be used under any circumstances. However, we will discuss how there can be both positive and negative forms of aggression. The former is actually a healthy form of being assertive while the latter is destructive to others and ourselves. Furthermore, within each of these two broad categories of aggression are various subtypes. Specifically, positive aggression can include Buddha Aggression, Righteous Indignation, Chivalric Aggression, and Masculine Aggression. Negative aggression can include

Flamethrower Rage and Misplaced Aggression. We will spend time defining each of these types of aggression later in the chapter.

# Positive and Negative Aggression

"Positive aggression" is a constructive force. It can be the emotional fuel that allows for goal-directed behavior, like sticking with a difficult task. For example, positive aggression is used by the artist who is caught up in the creative process and keeps working until the painting, sculpture, or other work of art is exactly the way it needs to be. This can also include a man who uses his aggression to help finish a physical challenge like a marathon, home improvement project, or other type of endurance test. Positive aggression can also help a man step into the competitive work of limited jobs and love interests and claim what he wants or needs. A man who finds his courage and stands firm in the face of weighty opposition is an example of a man who is displaying positive aggression.

The use of positive aggression is not all about serving the self; it is also present in moments of self-sacrifice. The fireman who runs into a burning building to save a baby needs this type of aggression. Likewise, when a man sees that someone he loves has been wronged by another, this aggression fuels the quest for justice and the drive to set things right. Also, when in the middle of a difficult patch within a committed relationship, it is the stuff that helps him endure and make appropriate concessions.

These positive forms of aggression are the basis for self-confidence, staying true to oneself, and the ability to protect those one loves. A man needs this functional form of aggression; it enhances his life and the lives of those he loves. One develops this positive aggression through the love and steady care of others. Good emotional care helps teach a man how to use his own power and gumption. The most effective learning involves being with a caregiver, leader, therapist, teacher, coach, or boss who allows him to experience positive aggression in healthy, constructive ways. These examples are preserved in a man's psyche and heart, and when it is his turn to own his personal power, he can draw on them.

Where aggression sours and becomes harmful is when it is born from chronic frustration and lack of emotional nurturance. This "negative aggression" is a destructive force that is potentially damaging to a man and others. The ultimate source of negative aggression is when people don't receive good emotional care in their lives on a consistent basis; it can leave a damaged spot inside the psyche and heart. Some in psychology embrace this interpretation of the origins and problems of aggression.

Making matters worse, the constrictive nature of the commandments causes the expression of this deep pain to be off-limits. Men learn to mask raw hurt through the more socially sanctioned but often unhealthy expressions of aggression; they can be too rough on the playground, in the office, or in the bedroom. It is important to note that expressing aggression in stereotypical ways, such as breaking things or getting into fights, doesn't soothe the deeper pain; in many ways it just aggravates it. In addition, this type of behavior leaves an emotional residual within the person and with others.

The commandments provide a way to mask the results of socially sanctioned forms of negative aggression, such as vulnerability, emotional hurt, and humiliation. However, to the untrained eye it may not seem as though any of these taboo emotions are actually being expressed. This approach is functional in a dysfunctional world of growing up male. This is a tricky way of disguising what is really going on while also getting emotions off his chest. Different forms of aggression do a fine job of masking these feelings; they can all get mashed into the secret shoe box. It is important to express emotions, even ones like frustration, anger, and hurt, but it needs to be done in ways that are consistent with healthy choices. Ultimately masking emotions can be confusing to everyone involved. As a partner or friend, you want to be able to decode what he is actually feeling when he is aggressive.

I realize that these differing notions of aggression may be new to some. In fact, the more positive form of aggression may be a stretch for some peoples' way of thinking. This is perhaps in part because we usually think of aggression only as acting hostile and violent—more like the negative form discussed above. And, of course, there is the history of violence that some people carry, having been on the other end of unhealthy aggression.

I have seen a number of male patients who initially present themselves as "nice guys" only to reveal later that they are intensely angry, in part because they feel constantly pushed around. When the whole story is uncovered, it is clear they are disenfranchised from their personal power; many feel others (friend, romantic partner, boss) take advantage of them and they are powerless to do anything about it. The formative years of these men usually involved a parent, often a father, who used intense negative forms of aggression in their child-rearing practices. The boy grows up and swears he will never be like his father. The boy then throws "aggression" and "power" into his emotional shoe box; both are emotionally compressed and often interpreted as being interchangeable. So being legitimately powerful feels tainted, as though he is following in his father's footsteps and being abusive to others, when, in fact, he is just being appropriately assertive. In these men's minds, being powerful always means being abusive. Sometimes the combination of societal and family issues makes us leery of positive power as a viable option.

I will freely admit that at times I have had a somewhat complicated relationship with authority. I laugh a bit too hard at irreverent comedies like *Family Guy*, look longingly at vintage Triumph motorcycles, and also have spent a fair amount of time sorting out viable versions of positive aggression. While I am not an "in your face" maverick, I value my own individuality a good deal and have a particular dislike for sweeping generalizations about "what I should do" based on someone else's dogma. This no doubt has its roots in my own background on multiple levels, from growing up as one of eight children, to my working-class roots, to having a special weakness for the underdog, and sometimes experiencing authority figures as less-than-ideal users of their own power.

When someone asked what I was doing at work, one of my favorite flippant jokes was to reply, "Trying not to work for the man!" It was a playful poke at authority, but there was some underlying edge revealed when I said it. Then, one day I was walking with a colleague, both of us the directors of our respective psychology programs. When he asked me what I had been up to lately, my pat answer about "the man" came out without a second thought. My colleague stopped, turned to me, and said, "But Chris, *you* are the man." "No, I am *not*," I said in utter horror and disbelief. "My whole life has been about railing against the man; what are you talking about?!" Then I realized he was right—that in some people's eyes, I was an authority figure. The upside of this was that it was an opportunity to further explore my own use of positive aggression.

Power and authority issues are usually revisited when the shoe is on the other foot and we are the ones who are now in charge, whether as a parent, teacher, or leader. Through considering my own personal matters from the past and their impact on me, I have learned to sort through when I am being my own man and using positive aggression as opposed to just rebelling and using the negative version of it. There are discernible differences. In its best light, my ongoing dance with authority has led me to challenge many things I have been told are absolute truths. To do this in a healthy way has helped carve out my own sense of individualism. When I am on track in this way, I am firmly rooted in my own truth.

On the other hand, in its worst light, my relationship with authority has sometimes led me to make bad choices in rebellion. This is not about adhering to my true self, but rather an unnecessary wrestling match with the powers that be. This negative aggression has sometimes caused me to miss out on what could have been good opportunities, and it also makes for an unnecessarily difficult ride. Finding my way through this maze has been a labor-intensive struggle at times.

Many men will find themselves in a similar boat about power issues, given that the commandments stress the notion that masculinity is based on increasing levels of authority and influence. The converse is also true: men feel demeaned when not in touch with the natural, human birthright of personal power. Many men are confused about the difference between unhealthy and healthy versions of power. Some of the specific types of power addressed below will clarify this. Let's take a look at a few examples of positive aggression and how these important tools can help. Remember, positive aggression deals with assertive behavior that benefits the individual and others.

# Types of Positive Aggression

## Buddha Aggression

Buddha Aggression is an enlightened use of positive aggression that involves confronting someone you care about who is making bad choices that may result in his ultimate self-destruction. Buddha Aggression gives you the gumption to deal with that person in a firm but caring way. You may have to confront a friend about a bad relationship decision, like having an affair, driving when drunk, or developing a dependency on pornography. This aggression is the fuel that gives a person both the courage to bring up and stay with a potentially difficult situation.

The assertive aspect of aggression is used in a compassionate way in order to discuss a situation in a straightforward manner. Conversations like this may begin with a comment such as, "I am worried about you because . . ." and "It upsets me to see you hurt yourself or others because . . ." The person receiving such feedback can react with gratitude and accept the message, or they can retort with a negative form of aggression. In either case, in the Buddha form of aggression, one does not get hooked into moving out of the caring, enlightened way of interacting. Sometimes the best endings that can be mustered in these conversations are wishing the person well and letting him know you will be there for him. The last chapter, on giving feedback to men, highlights the spirit and specific techniques involved with a Buddha-type positive aggression.

## Righteous Indignation

Righteous Indignation occurs when men who have been personally wronged desire to seek retribution. They are attempting to make the world seem right by seeking justice. This may appear in the office setting when someone has stolen your idea or claimed credit for your work. A direct confrontation may occur. It may also appear in a relationship when a wrong has occurred and a man seeks amends. This type of positive aggression is in bounds, justified, and appropriate.

Righteous Indignation involves a steady and firm confrontation with the wrongdoer. In the best situations, the seeker of justice may first confirm that the wrong has occurred and check out the intent of those who acted against him. The appropriate action can be determined at that point. If the slight was a misunderstanding, then the Righteous Indignation was the fuel that helped clear the air. If there is a more purposeful harm involved, direct words and actions may follow.

## Chivalric Aggression

This is the stuff of knights and cowboy tales. When someone a man holds dear is in danger or has been wronged, he sets out to settle the score, provide protection, or find justice on their part. This is a well-known theme in Hollywood plots where the tough guy sets out to right a wrong or shield a loved one. While Chivalric Aggression does not imply that gunplay or the death of the bad guy will soon follow, appropriate actions are taken to seek amends or redraw boundaries. This can range in modern times from being an advocate for your child at school when something inappropriate has occurred to upholding the honor of your partner. In all cases you are acting on the behalf of others in appropriate ways.

## Masculine Aggression

I realize that this particular version of aggression may sound a bit like the survival of the fittest. But this is the energy a man uses to go into the world of limited resources and lay claim to his share. This may include landing an account in the face of stiff competition or approaching and wooing a romantic interest. It may also involve having the gumption to stick to a difficult task like graduating college, running an endurance race, or committing to a personal ideal in the face of opposition. It may also involve a willingness to stick with tough commitments like being in therapy or facing the pain of the past. While this can appear in pseudoform as overblown bravado showcased by insecure knuckle draggers, most people—men or women—find the real deal a compelling form of self-confidence.

This type of positive aggression is born from healthy experiences with caregivers, peers, friends, and partners who gave the right balance of support and challenge. It gives a man the emotional fuel to step into the world. One of the best memories I have as a child involves being with my father one day when we were driving home alone. This was a rarity given that there were eight kids in my family. I was a little boy, no more than five years old, and I mentioned something about wishing I was old enough to drive. My dad had an old convertible sports car that he spent long hours trying to restore. It was still beat up for the most part, but it was a beautiful machine in my eyes.

To my surprise, my father pulled the car to the side of the road and told me I was going to get my chance to drive today. He said to hop into his lap. I was both excited and mortified. I grabbed the steering wheel and moved it back and forth to get the feel of it. I then quickly realized that my legs were way too short to "do the pedals." I said, "You will do the pedals, right?" He said, "Yes, I will do the pedals; you just steer the car." I remember experiencing a great sense of warmth and security that was so visceral it found its way inside my psyche and heart. Off we went!

Our short, little street seemed like it was miles long that day. I was having a big time steering while my father "did the pedals." Then, with a sense of panic, I remembered the driveway. I could steer straight down the street to avoid the curb, but to make that turn into the driveway . . . well, that was something I hadn't counted on doing. With that same sense of easing my anxiety, he put his hands over mine and said, "Here, I'll help if you need it, but I bet you can do it." Then we pulled into the driveway together.

That experience, and those like it with other encouraging people, both men and women, helped form a permanent part of my psyche. It acts as a reservoir of strength when I need it, allowing me to deal with anxious feelings when doing something that feels like a stretch or when pursuing my heart's desires. It also formed the basis for my ability to offer the same type of supportive challenges to clients and friends as an adult. The key things I learned from these life-changing occurrences is that we all need supportive, encouraging people in our lives; I will refer to these people as "guardians" in later chapters. The other thing is that we all need a steady balance of support and challenge, which ultimately is what really makes us strong.

Now that we've considered some of the positive forms of aggression, let's compare those with negative ones. Remember that these different types of negative aggression are usually harmful for everyone involved. They are also most likely created from chronic frustration, lack of support, and a depletion of emotional resources.

# Types of Negative Aggression

## Flamethrower Rage

Flamethrower Rage involves an intense reaction to a significant and usually painful situation in a man's life. Most men can sidestep many of the slings and arrows of life, but every once in a while, the layers of defenses can be pierced—especially if it hits close to the heart. This may include losing a job, feeling deeply discounted, finding out a spouse has been unfaithful, and so on. The aggression response can be rage. It may include yelling, name-calling, or, in the worst situations, violent acts such as fists through the wall, breaking things, or physically assaulting someone. All of these are unhealthy ways of expressing the intense feelings of hurt, belittlement, and humiliation.

Sometimes men don't know how to say they feel hurt. It seems a little too childish for some. And, as mentioned earlier, sometimes the support is not always in place to allow a man to work through these things. The commandments often hinder opening the secret shoe box to others in what would be a healthy way of working through these hurts. The commandments suggest men are not supposed to let anything affect them, but when they do, they should be self-sufficient enough to deal with it on their own. The balancing act in the male psyche is to let anger be the voice of emotional pain.

The intensity of the Flamethrower response also happens when a raw nerve is hit pertaining to emotional hurts that have built up over time and have not been dealt with. The level of intensity from past injuries and insults is fuel for the fire in the present situation and can be a marker for when professional help may be needed. Men who walk around angry all the time and express it in intense ways are carrying around a package that is destructive to self and others.

While this can be a very destructive form of negative aggression, if there is a silver lining to this cloud, it may be that if you can recognize this type of aggression for what it really is, and are patient enough and know how to handle it, the intensity will often give way to a softer appearance of vulnerability. (However, in its extreme forms, professional help is needed, and your own safety is paramount.) In some ways, it is a cry for help, reflecting internal broken parts. When handled properly, these situations can turn into potentially healing encounters. Some of the rawness can be soothed with empathy and understanding. We'll take a more in-depth look at this in Chapter 9, which is related to men's V Spots—their most vulnerable areas.

## Misplaced Aggression

Misplaced Aggression occurs when a man has experienced hostility directed toward him, and then he makes the choice to pass it on to another person as a way of discharging his own negative feelings for having been a target. Men learn about this trickle-down aggression while growing up.

Sometimes those who have been bullied learn to bully others. Or it may occur when caregivers or other authority figures misuse their power, setting up a continuing cycle for the male understudy to act in a similarly negative and aggressive way when it is his turn to play the leader. It may also appear when a boy feels like he is in a tenuous situation and about to go under from someone else's aggressive assault. He draws upon his man-training and employs the "duck, cover, and kick technique." This is a way of redirecting the focus of aggression onto another person. He can counter someone's verbal assault on himself by refocusing the attention upon someone even weaker.

This is a negative form of aggression on many fronts, because it does nothing to eliminate the hostility that circles the world. Instead, it is removed from your immediate sight and passed on to another. You may believe that because it has been passed on, it will no longer have an effect upon you, but as the old saying goes, "What goes around comes around." You have a bad day at work, so you're surly with your wife, who in turn is snappy with the children, who in turn are mean to the dog. The dog then chases the mail carrier, who in turn swears he is not coming back into your yard to be chased by a rabid dog, and thus leaves your winning Publishers Clearing House sweepstakes entry in his mail truck. You come home the next day and stare at the lawn, which now shows signs of a canine-mailman struggle, and you wonder why people can't be more civilized like you.

## Relationship Red Zone: Secret Decoder Ring for Aggression

| TYPES OF AGGRESSION | DEFINITIONS |
| --- | --- |
| Buddha Aggression | A compassionate aggression used to fuel a corrective confrontation with someone who is being self-destructive |
| Righteous Indignation | Setting the world right—fuels righting a perceived wrong done to you |
| Chivalric Aggression | Setting the world right—fuels righting a perceived wrong done to one you love |
| Masculine Aggression | Claiming what you need—fuels the ability to compete and persevere |
| Flamethrower Rage | Using aggression as a way of expressing hurt feelings |
| Misplaced Aggression | Using aggression as a way of covering potential vulnerability |

| TYPES OF AGGRESSION | ITS IMPACT |
| --- | --- |
| Buddha Aggression | Can help a friend, family member, or significant other get on the right track by changing self-destructive behavior |
| Righteous Indignation | Positive aggression—seeks justice for himself |
| Chivalric Aggression | Positive aggression—seeks justice for others |
| Masculine Aggression | Positive aggression—helps a man claim what he needs |
| Flamethrower Rage | Lets out feelings in a destructive, intense way—actual hurt feelings may go unrecognized |
| Misplaced Aggression | Passes on negative aggression to others |

# The Trouble with Sensitive Men

I remember watching the TV series *M.A.S.H.* when I was a kid. M.A.S.H. stood for Mobile Army Surgical Hospital, and the show chronicled the weekly wacky adventures of the doctors and nurses of the 4077 unit. There was Hawkeye and Trapper, the nonconformist surgeons, always at odds with the uptight regular army folks like Major Frank Burns and his girlfriend, Major Margaret "Hot Lips" Houlihan. Most of these episodes seemed to be fun-loving and free-spirited. However, the series began to change when mainstay characters began leaving the show.

And there was also Hawkeye's transformation: he had found his sensitive side. He was no longer defined as the woman-chasing drinker of homemade brew, but instead became an issue-raiser and the voice for sensitive men. Then it seemed that the actor who played Hawkeye, Alan Alda, had undergone a similar transformation. For some, he became a representative of the sensitive man movement of the 1970s.

And how about the Pittsburgh Steelers football player and tough guy Rosie Greer who appeared on TV commercials showing off his needlepoint? Of course, there was also the extreme of more gender-bending celebrities like David Bowie in his *Ziggy Stardust* fame. These changes were just a few of the new, more visible options that seemed to affect some men significantly. It gave them other role models to emulate besides the hardened John Wayne types. If nothing else, men began to reconsider traditionally held roles. Gender historians have noted that what ensued was a "men's movement."

Historians believe that numerous factors were involved in the inception of the men's movement. Included among these was the rise of the women's feminist movement, which led to a reexamination of traditional women's roles, which subsequently propelled men into reconsidering their notion of how to be a man. One of the changes was that in some circles, men had a little more leeway to be sensitive and claim they were proud of it. It showed they were enlightened and in touch with their feminine side.

But as with any social change, there can be a response, a backlash, if you will. The rejoinder was that sensitive men were "wimps." Where had all the real men gone? Who is going to fight wars and woo women in the old-school way with male bravado? Well, not sensitive men, that's for sure. Instead, they will attempt to seduce women by talking about their mother complexes and hoping their girlfriends or wives will take over where Momma left off. Some women's response to this was, "Hey, we like the newfound sensitivity and all but are not really looking for another boy to raise; any chance that's a club in your man purse?"

The trouble with sensitive men is that they get mistaken for being a bit leaky with their emotions. In reality, they are not necessarily the same thing. "Sensitive" means you are in touch with what you feel. You are even able to verbalize these things. By definition, you are also fairly attuned with what others—romantic partners, wives, friends, and children—feel. These are very good qualities that make for lasting connections. But where the confusion often occurs, and when being sensitive gets a bad rap, is when men have not developed an appropriate sense of mastery over their emotions. By the way, when we refer to "mastery over emotions" here, this is not employing the concept in the same way that the commandments often uses it, to direct men in cutting off the experience of bodily sensation and feelings. Instead, we refer to mastery in the area of emotions as having the appropriate levels of awareness and ease of use. But this is not effortlessly achieved.

We probably all know leaky folks, both men and women. They are folks who, much like the drinking glass that is cracked at the base, cannot contain their water even if they try. They get messy and leak all over the tables. And when others get too close, they leak all over them as well. Leaky people are emotionally untidy. Often, boundary issues are involved. Conversations with leaky vessel people can feel uncomfortable because there is often a crossing of the boundary of what is appropriate. On a first conversation, they may tell you of their deepest, darkest secrets or places of the most profound emotional wounding. They may discuss these topics in front of strangers or age-inappropriate children.

Often hooked to these disclosures is the wish that the person with whom they are conversing will be responsible for plugging up the leak in their vessel. The leaky people move from person to person, acting out this same drama. In our basic social skills training in kindergarten, we are taught that when people are in profound pain they either raise their hand or give the universal sign for choking, indicating something is amiss. Caring individuals respond to these signs, usually by giving reassurance or by offering aid in some way. But when encountered with individuals who are too leaky, too often, these caring types eventually feel put off or a bit used.

Now, some of you may be wondering, "Wait a minute. Haven't you been going on and on in this book about how people should be genuine and authentic, especially about how they feel?" Yes, I have, but there is a way to talk about who you are, even the most difficult parts, without doing it in a "leaky" way. Honest discussions in which you reveal yourself can be full of meaning and intimacy. You may share a part of yourself without the expectation that a person will step in to take care of you in inappropriate ways; you can talk about your feelings without trying to make someone else be accountable for them.

In healthy, established relationships, there are guidelines as well, such as a recognized reciprocity when talking about your day—the good, the bad, and the ugly; there is an ebb and flow, and each person gets a turn. And when one person is in especially dire straits, it is okay to have the talking stick for more than the normal allotted time. The couple, whether friends, family, or partners, knows that when they are in a bad place, the same courtesy will be afforded them. They try to establish an atmosphere where they surround the person with care, and the listening party does what they can to be caring and involved, but they are not ultimately responsible for what the other person does with this care.

When one is being leaky, the expectation is that the focus will always be on "me." Leaky people are so caught up in their pain that they tend to be self-absorbed and have trouble sharing in other people's joys and sorrows. Some examples of leaky men can be found in movies and TV shows. In the movie *Leaving Las Vegas*, Nicholas Cage plays a man who, having suffered several traumatic events, decides to go to Las Vegas to literally drink himself to death. During this time, he meets a woman (played by Elisabeth Shue) who happens to be a prostitute, and the rest of the movie chronicles their rather dysfunctional relationship. In a moment of supreme leakiness, Cage's character, accompanied by his girlfriend, is in a casino playing blackjack. When he asks for another drink, a waitress hints that maybe he has had enough. His response is to fly into a rage and begin yelling and screaming while he wreaks havoc upon the casino. It is only by his girlfriend's intervention that he is not literally thrown into the street by security.

Now, there may be several explanations for Cage's character's "leakiness"—too much drinking, too little self-control—but another notion is deeply embedded here: that his girlfriend is left with the responsibility of cleaning up his very big mess. He is a man with a self-destructive bent who, while he is drowning, elects to reach out and bring someone else down with him.

Though we should take the authenticity of all reality TV with a grain of salt, since we know that most of it is scripted for drama, they also provide striking examples of leaky people. Producers seem to ensure that each cast ensemble includes at least one such leaky person in order to spice things up, reek havoc on the stability of the rest of the cast, or provide a train wreck of personal drama viewers cannot help but watch. Some of these shows chronicle the adventures of childhood or would-be-stars struggling with forms of addiction on many levels: drugs, sex, fame, and fortune. Sometimes this includes following individuals making one self-destructive decision after another, affecting their relationships with others or their own general well-being. Even when more positive steps are taken, they are quickly undone or go off course.

What is also evident with leaky people is they are forever on a quest to find that thing that will plug the leak. Most people who have addiction issues are on this same mission. They want to find the thing that will make the pain go away. Most have tried to stop drinking, taking drugs, or acting out sexually, but when they try to stop, they come into fresh contact with the deeper underlying pain that drove them to the addiction in the first place. It is one of the reasons why relapses are so common; the original pain that cracked their vessel becomes intense again. Only by facing that pain and learning to make peace with it does the crack begin to seal. It is what eventually frees people from their bonds of servitude to their particular addiction.

So this applies to our discussion in that sometimes sensitive men get confused with leaky people because they have not yet mastered the skill of emotions, because wounds remain unhealed as a result of the commandments, or because they are in temporary crisis. Let's look at each of these. You may have gotten the impression that growing up male can leave a person ill prepared for the world of feelings, and that would be true. But men who make the commitment to broach this world in their adult lives go through a learning curve just like coming to terms with any new skill or task. You are not expected to get it squared away the first go-around.

Grown men trying to do this will make mistakes that appear to be leaky at first. This is normal and expected. In this process, they may not understand entirely what was clumsy about a particular emotional expression or interaction: "Hey, I was just getting in touch with my feelings, what was wrong with what I did?!" The image that may come to mind is a grown man who may be operating at the emotional equivalent of a much younger age, almost like a junior high schoolboy. And that is not a slight against him; after all, given the power of the commandments, he has some ground to make up for. One should expect to see this type of struggle until he has gained mastery over his emotions in a different, friendly way.

In an extreme version, leaky behavior can also reflect deep emotional damage as the result of emotional, physical, and sexual abuse. Not only have they missed out on so many of the emotional nutrients in childhood, but significant trauma was heaped upon them as well. Many of these people have an uneasy grasp on holding it together. They are prone to self-destructive coping skills built on aggression and aimed at themselves and others. In many cases, professional mental health services are needed.

Men may also be leaky when they are undergoing life-changing circumstances. This may include the death or loss of a spouse, child, or parent. It may also involve other major life changes: newly diagnosed diseases, disability, or career changes. These significant life changes are legitimate reasons to appear a little leaky when first discussing them. Just like the learning of a new skill has a growth curve, so does coming to terms with life when the deck is reshuffled in significant ways. A man's going to run across a stray wildcard now and then. To be leaky in these cases, for a time, is understandable. The challenge is to adapt to the new changes, making peace with them as much as possible. In some cases, meaning can even be found in significant losses.

## WAKE-UP CALL:
### Identify Leaky People

- Leaky people say inappropriate things at inappropriate times.
- There is an underlying message of "take care of me."
- Boundary issues are evident.
- The listener may feel used in conversations because there is no reciprocity.
- Leaky behavior may be due to crisis.
- Leaky behavior may be due to trying to master the learning curve of emotions.
- More permanent leaky people are missing significant emotional skills.

# Conclusion

One of the important things to keep in mind is that men can learn to live comfortably with their emotions. It's a skill set that takes practice, and part of the challenge is to become more comfortable with unmasking a wider range of emotions. To consider widening the circle can make many men uncomfortable at first. They bump up against the emotions deemed by their man-training as off-limits and subsequently use secondary emotions to cover what they actually feel. Often we can see the satirical edge of this real-life process in TV sitcoms, where men only learn about these taboo emotions after they get married and have kids. A man's tutor for his secret emotional life is often his wife.

However, whether on a sitcom or in real life, after so many emotional let-downs or blank stares with regards to what his wife wants from him, a man slowly realizes that if he wants a lasting relationship, he must go back to emotion school. While this may begin out of a sense of desperation like, "If I don't do some personal growth in this area my wife may leave me," often a man really does find that having a deep emotional life is rewarding in itself. Sometimes he even surprises his wife by exerting his newfound emotional knowledge, offering clever insights about the kids, friends, and family.

This whole progression can be a bit misleading when men begin to think they have crossed over into "a woman's world" by making friends with their emotions. They see the benefits of becoming more connected to their feelings but may also secretly wonder if they have become emasculated sell-outs. Of course, some of their male friends or colleagues may add a little fuel to this fire as well, sometimes offering more than good-natured pokes about his sensitive side coming into full bloom.

The truth is that neither gender has a monopoly on emotions. It is not a "man thing" or a "woman thing"—it is a human thing. Everyone is entitled to the full Crayola box of emotions. The tough part for many men (and also for those who accompany them on the journey) is that there is a distinct learning curve with emotions. Just like learning any new skill, most people grapple with the subtle and not-so-subtle nuances of fresh concepts. Most folks bumble and stumble before they catch on. Given that many men halted their education about the wide range of emotions long ago, there may be some catching up to do. The good news is that it can and has been done by many men.

# CHAPTER CUES

1. Emotions are not a "man thing" or a "woman thing" but rather a human thing.

2. People sometimes use secondary emotions to conceal (from themselves and others) how they feel.

3. Many men learn that sex and aggression are the only socially acceptable forms of emotion, sometimes used as secondary emotions.

4. Most forms of sex can have a positive and negative spin. What is essential to a good sex life is communication about what feels comfortable for both partners.

5. There are both positive and negative forms of aggression.

6. Positive aggression is the emotional fuel used to help a man go into the world and be his own man, as well as provide for and protect those he loves.

7. Positive aggression is developed through caring relationships that allow for the right balance of support and challenge.

8. Negative aggression does harm to oneself or others. It is created from chronic deprivation of emotional needs.

9. Leaky people are individuals who cannot properly regulate their emotions; they make inappropriate personal disclosures and attempt to make others responsible for taking care of them.

10. Sometimes men who are either learning to master emotions in a healthy way or going through a life transition can understandably appear leaky.

# 4

# Beyond the Body Armor:
# When Feelings Are Exposed

O nce, a male patient in his seventies began our session by telling me of his great love for the outdoors. He had spent a significant amount of time growing up in the "Great Northwest." He talked of skiing in the winter, hikes along the side of mountains in summer, and a litany of other ways he enjoyed the physical nature of his youth. The smile on his face slowly began to fade as he started checking off each one of these things he was no longer able to do. In fact, he came to our sessions using a walker, sometimes needing oxygen to help with his breathing, and found himself worrying about breaking a hip, as he contemplated his own mortality. As the sessions progressed, he wrestled with these thoughts and reactions, took a long pause, and said, "I guess because I am not able to do these things, it means I am not a man anymore."

When I was in high school, I remember talking with some of my buddies before football practice. We had just come from biology class and the lecture for the day concerned losing feeling in parts of the body where deep nerve damage had occurred. "You can't feel anything in those parts?" asked one of my friends, Fred. Fred was a big guy, played linebacker, and was physically tough as nails. He went on to become a Golden Gloves boxer. "That's what they say; you can't feel anything," I replied. Fred looked deep in thought and then later, when we were alone, he asked me if there was a way he could get some type of medical procedure in which he could purposely get nerve damage in both his arms. "Why would you want to do that, Fred?" I asked. "Well," he replied, "players from the other team would just bounce off my arms and I wouldn't ever feel any pain." "But Fred," I responded, "you wouldn't experience other things that felt good either." I could see I was wasting my words. Fred had drifted off into a dreamy world where he was imagining the trade-off of losing sensation in both of his arms in exchange for supposed mastery over his body. To him, it made perfect sense.

While the men in these two stories are vastly different in terms of age, both wrestled with the same fundamental aspect of masculinity: the relationship between the body and a man's understanding of his status as a man. The body is used as a tangible way of measuring if a man has achieved or is still able to sustain his masculine "mojo." From the first appearance of facial hair to the last tangible recollection of helping your now-grown children move furniture without concern for torn rotator cuffs, men use the body as an important barometer for their manliness. The status of the body in turn affects the psychology of being a man.

Anthropologist David Gilmore did a comprehensive study of masculinity across many cultures in the world. He concluded that in the vast majority of instances, masculinity is defined by the ability to achieve three major roles: protector, provider, and progenitor. We'll refer to them as the "Three Ps" for short. They refer to a man's ability to protect and provide for himself or those in his charge and father children. When a male is able to achieve these goals, he is granted the honorary title of "man." The successful fulfillment of the Three Ps is directly related to having a fully functioning "masculine body," one able to perform the tasks of a man.

The Three Ps draw heavily from the status of the body, signaling what can feel like the waxing and waning of being a man. For instance, reaching certain bodily milestones permits entry into the man club, which in turn affords special social rights and responsibilities that impact work and love.

Likewise, the anxiety of removal from the club awaits those unable to fulfill the corporeal challenges of the Three Ps any longer.

Men of all ages have lots of emotional investment in not only achieving the initial man status but also sustaining their own personal version of the Three Ps, something we will refer to as the "Man Checklist." This checklist details both entry and exit requirements of the man club. Special emphasis is given to items that represent the Three Ps lineup without which manhood seems impossible. The checklist is influenced by a man's own individual experiences: his relationship with his family, his upbringing, his romantic relationships, as well as his interface with the broader culture that dictates the creation of the commandments.

While there is some expected variability on what exactly appears on the checklist, certain themes originating from the Three Ps are to be expected. Some items are tucked into the corner of the mind, seen as taboo topics of discussion, though their power can still be felt. Others become the obvious and elaborated preoccupations that a man feels driven to achieve (or sustain), thereby safeguarding his sense of manhood. In either case, it takes a toll on him when he feels unworthy of joining the man club, falls short of the standard, or is no longer able to measure up.

## ▶ Toolbox Tip: The Man Checklist

This is an example of a hypothetical personal checklist rewritten throughout a man's life. Note that while some content changes, the underlying themes connected to the Three Ps are a constant presence. In some cases, items hit on more than one of the Three Ps themes of progenitor, provider, and protector. These are particularly emotionally loaded items to achieve or sustain. Also, the exact checklist requirement for the Three Ps is somewhat softened with age. While lowering the bar may not evoke the same level of being as "manly" as at the height of one's prowess, it does allow some sense of Three Ps manhood to be preserved.

## Personal Man Checklist as an Adolescent Boy

- Able to grow facial hair and shave regularly (*progenitor*).
- Get to third base with a hot girl at school (*progenitor*).
- Able to stand up to others. Develop "my guns" through lifting weights (*protector* and *provider*).
- Earn enough money to buy a car; girls will check me out (*provider* and *progenitor*).
- Don't let others see me sweat; no fear! (*protector* and *provider*).

## Personal Man Checklist as a Twenty-something Man

- Increased attention to sexual prowess; this can be expressed by marathon sex sessions or by having sex with multiple partners (*progenitor*).
- Lose that beer gut. Get ripped for summertime (*progenitor* and *protector*).
- Become a "do-it-yourselfer" renting or owning first home (*provider* and *protector*).
- Earn lots of money (including enough to buy a better car); girls will check me out (*provider* and *progenitor*).
- Be "man enough" to attract a long-term romantic partner. I am emotionally and physically strong; anything that does not match that persona must be stowed away out of view (*progenitor*, *provider*, and *protector*).

## Personal Man Checklist as a Middle-aged Man

- Still have twenty-something women flirt with me or find me attractive (*progenitor*).
- Still get an erection without the aid of Viagra (*progenitor*).
- Build up my IRA in lieu of declining physical prowess; still able to take care of my family financially (*provider* and *protector*).
- Do home improvement projects or subcontract aspects of them while I oversee (*provider* and *protector*).
- Earn enough money to buy a better car (preferably something foreign,

a classic car, or one with lots of horsepower); girls will check me out (*provider* and *progenitor*).

- Allow emotions to funnel into the body so no one sees me sweat; this includes worries about aging, providing for family, and any relationship problems with my spouse or kids. Emotional worries masquerade as health issues (*provider* and *protector*).

## Personal Man Checklist as a Postretirement-aged Man

- Still get an erection, period (any medical assistance acceptable) (*progenitor*).
- Maintain ownership of car and license (*provider* and *progenitor*).
- Want to feel useful to my children: help them with small projects around their houses, be a source of information about buying or owning a home, and so on (*provider* and *protector*).
- Years of being emotionally out of touch have taken a toll on mind and body; try not to show others when it hurts (*provider* and *protector*).

If one examines the Three Ps closely, it becomes apparent that a man places a great deal of emphasis on these abilities early in his manhood career. In fact, they are by definition the ones that grant him admission into the man club. The central problem is that the world of men, young and old, seems governed largely by a younger man's checklist of what constitutes masculinity. This emphasis on youth culture is built into the Ten Commandments of Growing Up Male.

Men strive to move through physical and social rites of passage as quickly as possible in order to achieve man status, or at least the young man's definition of it. As we will see in Chapter 8, a rite-of-passage approach when used wisely can potentially provide ways of helping make life transitions. However, this same formula is often skewed when applied to today's notion of men and masculinity. These behaviors, as they pertain to the body, can include the physical aspects of having gone through puberty, growing body and facial hair, developing muscles, voice change, and so on—all things of great concern to younger men and those susceptible to a hypermasculine bravado.

The rite continues in a social context involving the first drink (or drunk), sexual experience, or the successful completion of some test of endurance or physical pain. These are tangible signs of having achieved a hardy, manly physique, though these tests of manhood can also turn into trials of needless abuse. In more advanced versions of the rite, the focus is on mastering all things painful. This includes the realms of physical and emotional pain. When no one ever sees you sweat, you have taken a big step toward becoming a man. "No fear" bumper stickers and the like seem to convey a message of being beyond the normal realm of human emotion. We could extend these notions further as a man becomes the progenitor of children through his potency, or, in a more symbolic way, successful in his career through the sweat of the brow. In both of these cases, the emphasis is not necessarily on the responsible use of mojo, but just making sure you have some, regardless of potential costs.

Beyond the notion of man status (am I a man or not?), the checklist also speaks to what degree of manliness one possesses. The dreaded "short man's disorder" and endless competitions that smack of "is yours bigger than mine?" figure into the preoccupation of many men of all ages. The "bigger is better" mentality shows up in true Darwinian fashion as men attempt to be the biggest, most powerful ape on the block. The underlying belief is that enhancing the body sometimes to exaggerated proportions means becoming more of a man.

Achieving a "man-up" in terms of the body may in turn feel like an automatic upgrade as a protector, provider, and progenitor, making a man feel more competitive on the open markets of work and love. No doubt, the advertising masterminds on Madison Avenue play to this equation, encouraging men to look deep into their wallets when actual physical upgrades are not so easily achieved. Marketing a new product with the right masculine edge often involves adding a little extra muscle, making it bigger, stronger, and faster.

Or, if a male feels unsure in his body with romantic interests or at work, then maybe there are ways to psychologically offset these feelings of uncertainty. A sports jersey, the right SUV, or an oversized stainless steel outdoor grill are but a few of the ways to gain some relief. After all, commercials say he becomes more of a man by owning these things, and after a while, he may start to believe it himself. Many males strive to "man-up," and why not? The commandments speak to the dual-edge nature of man status: untold riches lie in store for assuming the role of a "real man" (even if some of that requires taking on a false persona), while one can feel like being a second-class citizen for not being man enough.

There are a few other points to consider about the Three Ps and the personal checklist. First, with regards to the Man Checklist, there is not a definable endpoint indicating when the status of masculinity is assured forevermore. Rather, as with the natural course of aging, some of the items on the list become out of reach and are no longer possible, and then one's status as a man can feel in jeopardy. A strategy to combat this worry is to achieve an approximation of one or more of the Three Ps in hopes that it will be enough. So if a middle-aged man can't have the same sexual prowess he once did as a twenty-something, the next best thing is to find a little help in pill form—not exactly the same, but close enough for now. That is, until one or more of the Three Ps is completely extinguished. What then?

Also, what is particularly interesting is the lack of additional male roles that follow the initial admission requirements for entering the man club. You just cross the barrier into manhood and stop growing or evolving. Shouldn't there be a next step(s), something more to strive for, like a "mature masculinity" beyond the entry level of the Three Ps? Also, there are other aspects of the checklist that speak of "mastery" over the body that can actually lead to an unhealthy disconnection from the natural birthright of experiencing physical sensation and emotion. Not feeling things does not imply competency, much less mastery in life. Part of a rewarding life includes allowing various sensations to be experienced in the body; the goal should not be to become numb to every other emotion besides sex and aggression by the age of thirty. One of the side effects of trying to do such a thing is that the volume on all emotions slowly gets turned down over time, which may result in a condition called "alexthymia"—an inability to register and express feelings of all kinds. Those in such a state have lost touch with and control over their emotions and physical bodily sensations.

From this brief introduction, we can see that men's emotions and bodies are complex, interrelated, and potentially misunderstood. Here is a brief summary of the themes that have been touched on so far:

- There is a personal Man Checklist based on the Three Ps (protector, provider, and progenitor) that emphasizes tangible markers of masculinity, each of which centers on the development of the body and its prowess.
- A skewed rite-of-passage mentality is often applied to masculinity where men are taught to master their bodies by not feeling physical sensations or emotions.
- The Man Checklist is confusing and limiting because it emphasizes only a young man's notion of masculinity, yet it governs men across the life span.

## The Darker Side of a Man-up

*Theme No. 1: There is a personal Man Checklist based on the Three Ps (protector, provider, and progenitor) that emphasizes tangible markers of masculinity, each of which centers on the development of the body and its prowess.*

A clear perspective on the "bigger is better" mentality can be easily lost. Men can operate under the notion that being the biggest, most powerful ape on the block, in whatever symbolic form, will afford them the choice of romantic partners or other special social and financial considerations. Today's masculine misconceptions and the media coverage that reinforces them do much to propel these notions as a surefire guarantee for everlasting happiness, rather than an adolescent fairy tale to be debunked.

For instance, in relationships, this formula is sometimes referred to as the "social exchange theory," where men and women each bring something to the relationship negotiation table in hopes of getting something in return. One definition of a "trophy husband" is based on his storehouse of material riches, which can in turn lure a "trophy wife," usually prized because of her physical beauty. To say this arrangement isn't operative in today's society would be inaccurate. In fact, much of traditional masculine culture promotes these notions in music videos, commercials, and sports venues. It seems that the target to shoot for in order to ensure a man's everlasting happiness involves muscles and money. Having more of each would mean he himself is more; his value as a human being would increase.

The downside of this faulty equation is only realized when he reaches the apex of his physical or financial prowess and either he or his wife discovers that, while it is nice to look good and cover the bills, these things cannot ultimately make you happy. There needs to be something that is more permanent and less conditional if a sense of healthy well-being is to be sustained across a lifetime. In failing to discover this deeper truth, many men may feel compelled to alter the limits of their bodies far beyond their original design by employing "training enhancers." To man-up may also involve other symbolic means like increases in horse- and manpower, or worse, preying upon others. All of these are done in the name of increasing perceived man status.

Sadly, boy's sports culture, as well as school and gang violence, draws upon these same formulas of social climbing and masculine compensation. After all, learning to be a man, even if it is a distorted image, takes years to develop. Here we see the darker side of the man-up. For instance, some research shows that the physiques of boys' action figures have undergone dramatic changes in the last thirty years. Take *Star Wars* figures as one example. It seems that Luke Skywalker has been hitting the gym pretty hard in the years following the early 1970s films; even G.I. Joe's biceps have grown from about fourteen to more than twenty-six inches in real-life measurements. Other action figures are even more pronounced, some featuring the real-life equivalence of thirty-two inch biceps! What this suggests is that boys can be exposed to the fallacy that bigger always means better and that bigger improves their standing as a man, even from a very young age.

The darker side of man-ups can also involve ways to express emotional frustrations in the form of overly aggressive fantasy play. Action figures and video games are a few routes that a boy may take to gain a new, more grown-up role or identity, sometimes feeling larger and more powerful than he actually is. This fantasy technique, truth be told, is not inherently bad. In fact, in its proper measure, it can be a helpful part of a boy safely stretching and practicing for his role as a grown-up. The development of a masculine presence is not solely dependent on the mastery of various viable forms of healthy aggression, but it helps. This process goes astray when he pushes the boundaries of healthy aggression and gets stuck in this exaggerated form of play, or when the boy must slip deeper into the fantasy world as his only means to offset the events of the real day. For instance, he transforms into a he-man in private after a day of feeling less-than in the presence of others, whether with peers, coaches, teachers, parents, family, or friends.

Remember, negative, unhealthy aggression and its subsequent uses are often born from a lack of nurturing and support. Negative, aggressive play-acting becomes a way of balancing things in the psyche when a man feels adrift or when it does not feel safe enough to grant others access to his inner realm. In the extreme, he learns to make others suffer in his imaginary world as he himself has and still does in the real one. He slowly becomes desensitized and impervious to the pain of others. "Why should I care?" he thinks, as he assumes his supervillain persona. "No one cares about me."

To understand the inflated form of the body in terms that are more symbolic is the real challenge. Sometimes these complex notions are interrelated, woven tightly together to form a protective body armor for a man. This can be a figurative or literal way to defend against deeper insecurities, not measuring up to the commandments, and having a convenient stowaway compartment for things he would rather not feel. In severe situations, masculine uncertainty reflects much deeper issues, ones where the core notion of worth as a human being is damaged. In these cases, not addressing deeper issues leaves few choices besides employing a string of never-ending coping skills without really addressing anything that is damaging or dysfunctional.  The most deadly combination is when personal damage is both perceived as irreversible and deemed completely off-limits to others. This becomes, as psychologist Dr. Glenn Good suggested, a male double bind, where you are damned if you do seek help, because it is against traditional expectations for being a man, and damned if you don't because you suffer in silence. Given the liabilities of the situation, some may conclude that the next best thing involves a buildup of impenetrable body armor. A man thinks this will be able to protect the injured psychic areas within. The boy, or later, the man, surmises, "No one can touch that broken part of me when I am ten feet tall and bulletproof." In theory, this plan guarantees the wearer unwavering safety, only to reveal later, at the onset of male depression or in more extreme situations like school shooters and professional wrestlers taking the lives of others and then themselves, that it does not hold true. In those instances, we can assume that boys/men are placed in direct contact with the intolerable psychological threats that can only, at best, be temporarily shielded.

## ▶ Toolbox Tip: The Body as an Emotional Defense

As we will see in the chapters that follow, if a man desires to live comfortably in his own skin, it is necessary to reexamine the items of the secret shoe box that never fit peacefully within—the things that rumble and thrash, echoing the worries and pains of the past. For some men, both the marker and eventually the doorway into this process lie within the exploration of the symbolic messages the body is attempting to simultaneously send and conceal. To pull back the symbolic protective body armor means revealing the more genuine human being concealed beneath. This may include seeing how an überpowerful exterior is actually employed as a means to cover previously unseen and vulnerable areas. A gruff manner, big muscles, or badass wardrobe may be used to protect against all incoming assaults or to camouflage damage already done before he suited up.

## Mind/Body Connection in Men

Sometimes the body is used as a combination of psychological defense and punching bag in dealing with more underlying emotional issues. As you might guess, these approaches are not always helpful and can lead to some damaging consequences, such as high blood pressure and heart disease, which can result from the anger-driven Type A personality; other times, emotional conflicts aggravate already existing medical conditions. Unresolved troubles may also masquerade as medical symptoms, such as when chest pain is really anxiety. The second theme of this chapter explores the mind/body connection, which for some men is actually a disconnection.

*Theme No. 2:* A skewed rite-of-passage mentality is often applied to masculinity where men are taught to master their bodies by not feeling physical sensations or emotions.

I used to work at a community clinic where part of my responsibilities included training medical students. One of the things I tried to impress upon them was the way the mind and body worked directly together. Some students, trained in the medical arts, forgot to consider other, more emotional/mental factors when making a medical diagnosis; they treated the mind and body as very separate entities, as if one had no influence on the other. Sometimes a gentle reminder was needed that life events such as stress, job situations, divorces, and so on could worsen or create physical troubles.

But the connection between mind and body should not only be stressed in medical training, but also in everyday living. For instance, the mind's reaction is sometimes led by the body's faltering condition. When you feel physically sick, the emotional part of you can also fall prey to the body's influence and suffer. This is the body taking charge and literally leading the mind—but being physically sick does not mean you have no say over your emotional response. I experienced this firsthand while doing part of my internship at a cancer wellness center, where the core treatment philosophy involved dealing honestly with emotions. Many of the people I encountered within that community focused on engaging all of life right up until the very end. Some even spoke of the "gift of cancer" because of the many life lessons it taught them about living, loving, and reprioritizing their lives.

Some research suggests that this method of the mind leading the body may be an effective aid in combating cancer and other illnesses. After all, chronic emotional states like depression and anxiety can cause certain chemical changes in the body. It is like putting extra miles on a car. We all know people who have gone through a difficult emotional period and suddenly seem to age overnight. What we can do to reduce the load of stress helps us both emotionally and physically. This mind/body emphasis underscores the importance of how we function in a holistic way, each aspect impacting the other for better or for worse.

How does this mind/body business figure into our discussion about men and emotions? It is important to allow an easy flow between having emotional reactions and actually being able to register them in the body. The training many men experience is exactly the opposite of this healthy equation: emotions are mastered by keeping them in check or, even better, not acknowledging they even exist. To aid in this, some see the body as a great storage shed for all that unwanted emotional stuff. If this baggage is stowed out of sight, they start believing that it does not really exist; but eventually, the resulting clutter can take a toll physically as well as emotionally.

Since the early days of psychology, there have been a number of psychologists who recognized what Freud suggested about dammed-up, conflicted emotions: they have to go somewhere. If conflicts are not freely discussed and worked through at a conscious level, they can pop up in a number of symbolic and unexpected ways, like the guilt-ridden soldier coming back from battle who suddenly develops paralysis in the hand that fires his rifle. Or, in more everyday occurrences, a man may not discern that he develops bodily symptoms like headaches, heart palpations, or tension in his chest after unacknowledged anxiety about his job or a fight with his wife.

When men are too far out of touch with their own emotions, pressure may begin to heighten. As these unacknowledged emotions build, sometimes intense physical sensations begin to express the feelings that are stirring. Men who follow this pattern end up in the emergency room, thinking they are having a heart attack because of chest pain, light-headedness, and a racing pulse. Their wives and kids gather around their bedside waiting for the worst possible news, until the doctor comes in and reports a clean bill of health. "It was just anxiety," he says. "You might want to go talk to someone about the stress you're under."

In these cases, when emotional conflict is not dealt with directly, the body's reactions can act as an emotional vent. Under times of distress, bodily symptoms flare up, allowing some expression of the real emotional conflict that lies beneath. This technique of emotional venting can afford some temporary relief, but in the long term, it can be pretty problematic. A man can begin to mix up physical sensations with his emotions, not knowing which is which. For some men, this results in an overriding sense of truly not knowing what they feel. To the outside observer, they also can mistakenly label emotional symptoms as physical ones.

To understand emotional venting and men's relationship with emotion and their bodies, we must draw upon the secret shoe box concept discussed in Chapter 2. That most private area of a man's life needs to respond in step with the ever-changing complexities of his life. Part of what gives the secret shoe box breathing room and sustained order is making sure a man has good access to its contents and is able to share them with caring others. If this does not happen in appropriate ways, things begin leaking through the walls; sometimes issues end up expressing themselves in the body because there is nowhere else to go. However, there are limits even to this approach.

A patient I worked with once had chronic back pain from an injury.

While he had surgery and was on pain medication, he was able to function under normal circumstances. However, when his life got hectic, he would get really down on himself for not being able to work harder. This was not a friendly, internal pep talk; rather, he belittled himself in an unmerciful way for not being able to do more, back injury or not. Of course, this way of trying to motivate himself was too harsh. He actually ended up getting so stirred up by all his internal workings that his back paid the price; he ended up having to miss work for a week. During that week off, he became so medicated that he had little choice in taking a break from being so hard on himself, and his actual physical condition subsided. Maybe it does not have to go to that extreme for men to find some relief.

You need to be able to appreciate that these patterns of becoming separated from the body take time to develop. Some men may take pride in their disconnection, since expressing emotion is perceived as a sign of weakness. After all, a central theme of the commandments places an emphasis on not letting things like pain or emotional or physical issues stop you. Sometimes this is taken to the extreme, and men begin to experience a domino effect of phasing out various levels of emotional awareness and sensation over time. When a man shuts down emotionally, he may experience a false sense of being stronger, but what has really happened is that he has become numb to the emotional sensations that are a natural part of being human. Being strong has little to do with *not feeling*. Instead of not feeling, a man can learn to reengage with his emotions and body, but this takes time.

If the man in question has become numb to his emotions, sometimes the remaining bodily sensations are the primary way he experiences things. He may secretly realize he only really feels things when they are associated with the body, like working hard, eating, drinking, and having sex. In some cases, even these bodily sensations begin to feel dulled over time. At some point, he may sheepishly reveal to someone that his normal state of being is numbness. "Why is it you can't feel things?" a loving partner, friend, or family member may ask upon discovering his sensation status. In a panic, the same person may try to prompt him back into the feeling world through an assault on his emotions. This approach, while well meaning, usually results in the opposite of the intended effect: the man will most likely withdraw further after a befuddled attempt to appease you.

When these issues come up again, or if you make it your mission to get him to feel again, he may do anything to stop the onslaught of being under the "emotional interrogation lamp." "Sure, yes, I think I am feeling something now . . . yes, I am sure of it . . . don't know what it is . . . but I think it is an emotion . . . is that enough for today?" The commandments pressure men to be competent in all things, even in areas where they are not. Part of their man training is to cover up those areas. It can be shaming to not be good at something and have others hover over you. The message they hear is "You are broken; what is wrong with you?"

## Reestablishing the Mind/Body Connection

Sometimes a man has to reestablish his emotional connections by first getting in touch with his physical ones. It is almost the reverse order from what you would expect, but his body may be the most viable place to start, because he still has sensations there, and when properly explored, these sensations may lead to a (re)connection with other aspects of himself, like emotions.

In this process of turning up the volume on physical sensation and then emotional attentiveness, there can be a lot of initial static, resulting in confusion. He may have to learn to differentiate between what feels like indigestion and actual emotional upset. Once I worked with a man who was referred for chronic anxiety that sometimes manifested itself as chest pain. He had been disconnected from his emotions for some time, using alcohol to help self-medicate when he felt nervous about work or relationships. He came into treatment because he thought he had suffered a heart attack but found out it was actually a panic attack.

We worked together, trying to get him more connected to his emotions through tracing the sensations he felt. He initially thought he was just stumbling onto "tangents," but what he was really doing was discussing the underlying cause of his body's symptoms, the things that bothered him. This man was used to dumping his emotions into his body, which served the purpose of being a vessel for uncomfortable things he would rather not experience.

As we talked about "tangents," many of which involved both past and present-day troubles, and sorted them out, his chest pain and anxiety level got better. However, he noted that the chest tightness had not gone entirely, and in one session, he began talking about trouble with his wife. He sometimes did not feel supported by her, and as he was discovering—beneath all the layers of former numbness—this was upsetting to him. When he did not acknowledge this to himself, his chest hurt—believe it or not, right over his heart. Sometimes the emotional conflicts can symbolically manifest themselves. On the one hand, they can be indirectly expressing the underlying problems, while on the other, they can also be viewed as an invitation to delve deeper into a more real relationship between the mind and the body.

A mind/body journal may be helpful for reestablishing the link between a man's sensations and emotions. Keeping a journal is very simple to do. He can carry around a pocket-size notebook and record situations where he notes his body is speaking to him. In one column, he can write down the actual event that happened, like, "Upset stomach," "Chest pain," "Head- and backache." In the next column, he can write down any emotional or mental event that preceded the bodily sensation and may have impacted it: "Chewed out by the boss," "Fight with wife," "Argument with coworker." In the last column, he can record any hint of an emotion that was present, even if he is not sure he can express them exactly. He may feel like he is pulling at threads at first. After a week or two of doing this, however, he may actually see more of a connection between bodily sensations and the appearance of emotions.

## ▶ Toolbox Tip: Mind/Body Journal

| BODY SENSATION | PRECEDING EVENT | FEELINGS |
|---|---|---|
| Headache | Chewed out by boss but couldn't say anything back; thought I might lose my job | Angry; frustrated; maybe embarrassed? |
| Upset stomach | Fight with wife about her wanting to buy "expensive" new baby furniture | Misunderstood; alone |
| Chest Pain | Discussion about having first child that did not go well; did not say all that I was thinking because she (wife) looked so happy about being pregnant | Anxious (can we afford new furniture now?) Worried (Will I be a better parent than my father who was never around?) |

You can support him by letting him bounce these experiences off you and helping him sort through what he felt. Mind you, at times, and depending on the level of numbness that is present, it may feel like you are helping your third grader with his foreign language homework. This is an area that may be very new to him, so enter into this exercise with a spirit of patience; fight the knee-jerk reaction to cajole him, even on occasions that may not make a lot of sense. "You felt what? Well, that is ridiculous; you're a grown man, for God's sake!"

Also, on occasion *you* may be the item on his list that evoked an emotional response. You may not like this or agree with him, but your job is to validate what he felt (of course, this type of exercise lends itself well to working on communication in the relationship as well). Remember, this is about helping him feel things again. He may have misperceived a situation that led to an emotional reaction, and by bringing it up, you have the opportunity to clear the air. There certainly may be bumps along the road with this exercise when you come up as an item on his list. In these cases, he may be testing you to see if he's emotionally safe with you. There may be other feelings he is discovering, ones toward you that he wants to discuss. While this may not feel so great at first, the upside is that it will pay off in the long run because his ability to *feel* will enhance your relationship as well. It allows for a fuller realm of feelings toward others, including you.

### ▶ Toolbox Tip: Nonsexual Massage

Another way of trying to get your partner in touch with his bodily sensations is by giving him a nonsexual massage. The rules are established from the outset that this is not a form of foreplay; it is about being more in touch with bodily feelings. If it quickly turns into sex, then the purpose of this is defeated. He probably already pushes a lot of emotions into his body during sex. This needs to be something different.

The massage can be full body or focused on one specific part, like feet, neck, or back. Be creative; set a relaxing mood by using candles, music, or massage oil. All he needs to do is focus on how his body feels. This can be uncomfortable for some men at first. It means they are letting their guard down and opening themselves up to body sensations, and eventually, feelings.

Some of you may be thinking, "Hey! I would like a nonsexual massage, too. Why does he get all the fun?!" Well, that is the upside of this exercise—he can play, too. Set an egg timer and take turns, or assign your own days of the week. Part of his work is to be inside his own skin as he touches you. He can learn a lot by *giving* a nonsexual massage as well, such as learning that bodily sensation does not always equal sexual arousal.

### ▶ Toolbox Tip: Awkward Moments

In this process of helping a man become more connected to his bodily sensations, and in turn his underlying emotions, a romantic partner needs to be especially prepared for the unexpected. Turning up the volume on feeling emotions has the tendency to stir up old emotional wounds, some of which you may not have known existed. In fact, you may unexpectedly discover that some of this stuff is the reason why he learned to become disconnected from emotions in the first place: because it hurt.

Many well-meaning partners find themselves struggling in such moments, when they get exactly what they have been asking for: their man actually begins feeling things. However, sometimes this may not appear in a neatly packaged form, nor is it in keeping with how he normally "does" emotions, both of which can lead to a number of reactions, including shock and discomfort. While "Holy crap, what do I do now?" or "You weren't suppose to have that intense of a reaction until I finish reading that book!" may be only a few of your responses, it is really important that these not be damaging moments for either person involved. He should not feel prematurely overexposed, and you don't want to feel like you have failed him. Chapter 11, on being a guardian, goes into detail about how to handle situations like these. For right now, an acknowledged preemptive caveat between you and your partner is sometimes warranted. Something like "I am going to give you this massage, and let's just go slowly with the hope that you are registering these sensations, which will also help you become more aware of other things, like your emotions. Now, if you start feeling things that you don't understand and I don't know how to handle, let's make a deal to take a break; neither one of us has to master this all in one massage."

## When the Body Fails Us

There is yet another way that a man experiences his bodily sensations. It is not as a sign of male insecurity or a psychological defense. Sometimes there is real joy in being in the body. He feels exhilarated by the pleasures of physical work and exercise, the simple enjoyment of a hard day's work, a good cup of coffee on a cold day, or going for a walk in the woods to see the deer jump impossibly high. All these things can cause the blood to pump through his veins, making a man know he is alive. We cannot overlook moments of gentleness in the body either, expressions of tenderness, whether that is making love or holding another that is beloved. These sensations become indelibly pressed into the flesh as body memories. All of these and more reflect a healthy way to enjoy the body. For many men it is not only a symbol of prowess and maleness, but a site of pleasure and sensation. There is a legitimate sense of loss when the body seems to fail to register and react as it once did.

I was diagnosed with Ménière's disease when I was a few years shy of forty. While there are far worse medical complications, this one can be unpleasant. It involves loss of hearing and balance, tinnitus (ringing in the ear), migraines, mental fog, fatigue, and perhaps worse, bouts of unpredictable and pronounced vertigo. Sometimes I would be sitting in a meeting or teaching a class and get the sensation that we were all on a boat rocking up and down on the waves of the sea. Sometimes the waves would gently touch the sides of our ship, and other times, they crashed against it. In bad situations, the "man overboard" sign needed to be posted as I dealt with the boat spinning in circles, leading to what could be hours or days of vomiting and disorientation. While it is not fatal, Ménière's disease is often progressive and difficult to control; some who have it end up on disability from its effects. Attempts at controlling symptoms include various medications and surgeries. My treatment involved undergoing procedures that traded permanent disruption of balance and complete hearing loss in my left ear for more control of vertigo. One of the upsides of such procedures was that I didn't hear myself snoring anymore if I slept with my good ear to the pillow. But I did wonder if my days of exercising, making furniture, doing home improvement projects, and working with my hands were gone. Living in my body was very connected to my own sense of masculinity. It was also the way I stayed in touch with my working-class roots, and, in some ways, using my body was when I felt most alive.

Shortly after this diagnosis, I was at a writer's museum in Dublin, Ireland, reading about Jonathan Swift, the author of *Gulliver's Travels* and fellow Ménière's patient. "They say he went mad from it," the helpful museum attendant said. "Really?" said another one, "I thought that was a disease that only little old ladies got." Neither comment prompted much hope in me that there would be a simple or smooth transition.

For men who have seen their bodies as a source from which their sense of manhood emanates, or simply as a center of real pleasure, there is the need for real adjustments when it begins to change. For instance, does it mean you are not tough anymore because you can't do the things you used to? And if you are not physically as tough as before, does that also somehow strip away your sense of masculinity? Or is it as the patient mentioned at the beginning of this chapter confided to me when noting the ever-growing list of things he was unable to do from his youth, "Well, I guess that means I am not a man anymore"? These important questions reflect the third theme of men and their bodies:

**Theme No. 3:** *The Man Checklist is confusing and limiting because it emphasizes only a young man's notion of masculinity, yet it governs men across the life span.*

The commandments confirm there is a definable checklist of masculine behaviors that when fulfilled allows one to cross the threshold into the bona fide world of manhood. Given what we have noted so far about the commandments, achieving such a status is itself a daunting task. Adding to the difficulty of this situation is that one's man status is not permanent. When unable to carry out the prerequisite manly duties any longer, the membership card is revoked. For some men, items are sadly checked off as they feel their sense of masculinity slip away. While this list does have some variability by person, and not all items carry the same weight, there can be specific ones that seal the deal, indicating membership in the man club is over.

I consulted with a medical patient once who had spent his entire life working as a mechanic. He was by all accounts knowledgeable, hardworking, and a tough old guy, but his medical condition made it impossible to hold his tools for any normal length of time anymore. His wife brought him into the medical clinic, thinking he was depressed. He talked about how he had worked with his hands all his life and how that defined who he was. He did show signs of being depressed, but to be more accurate, he was experiencing a sense of bereavement. The man was losing a central part of who he was, so of course he was going through an adjustment period as he tried to come to terms with his new reality.

I am also reminded of famous writer, journalist, and adventurer Ernest Hemingway. He was a man who epitomized the traditional notion of masculinity in the twentieth century. He was a fighter, hunter, drinker, and lover of women. As legend goes, he woke up one morning and found his pants did not fit as they used to, went into a closet, and shot himself. I first heard this story when I was a young man and wondered a long time about it: "Why would a man shoot himself because his pants didn't fit anymore?" To take this story, or those like it, at complete face value would be far too simplistic. One of the things I have learned in the years since first encountering this story is the complex nature of people. Attempting to encapsulate another's life or demise as a sound byte does not do proper justice to the person or surrounding circumstances. Such attempts try to make sense of a difficult situation by pointing to the prominent symbols around which we construct the core definitions of others.

This same reduction process occurs on a more personal level when we are the ones in transition. People often discover firsthand that simple generalizations do not neatly capture the complexity of the situation. If people ask and really want to know what is going on, it might take a little while to explain. When those symbols that carry personal meaning such as physical health, relationships, or life roles begin to fade or are stripped away, they can cause an erosion of the most basic notion of identity. Losing core pillars of selfhood would be hard enough, but many people find these symbols are ultimately tied to other self-definitions, creating a domino effect of change. People are left wondering, "If I am not *this me* anymore, than who am I?" The number of factors—such as the level of available support, additional stressors in one's life (past and present), and how many losses have to be negotiated—will ultimately dictate how well one can transition to a new identity.

Into this complex maze, we begin to grapple with the reality of our own eventual aging. I believe that a man's sense of masculinity does not have to be stripped away as he ages, but instead could be of some aid in this process of readjustment. Kirk Douglas, Hollywood legend, star of more macho man movies than you can count, and father to Michael Douglas, appeared at the Oscars a few years ago, shortly after having suffered a stroke. He was there to accept a lifetime achievement award, which was presented to him by his son. Though his speech was notably slurred, he showed remarkable zest and vigor. HBO subsequently produced a documentary on the Douglas father-son relationship. One of the most interesting parts of it was that his wife said the years since his stroke had been Kirk's happiest. Isn't that amazing? But how could that be? A man who had made his name in Hollywood playing a Viking, cowboy, gangster, and soldier, and was now physically limited, was at the happiest point in his life. One answer may be found in the interview. She said he had nothing left to prove. He also seemed to transition to a different way of relating with his family that was more connected and less like the characters he played in the movies.

Sometimes the supreme teacher is loss, inviting us to face the inevitable impermanence of all things. Without hitting this roadblock, we would not willingly come to accept the inevitable—that we all age and must face our own demise. This new assault on consciousness can come in the form of a startling wake-up call when we suffer sudden changes in health, as well as the gradual decline that accompanies normal aging. I have spoken with a number of men who have had their lives disrupted due to health issues; in the best of cases, it can lead to better life choices and an enhanced quality of life. However, this does not mean that in every case all that was lost can be somehow miraculously restored. It has more to do with acceptance and adjustment. I am convinced that every change in our lives has the potential to yield meaning, including gaining a deeper understanding of the world, human nature, and especially ourselves.

All of these changes can become true gifts for a man, though at first they appear to be anything but treasures. The trick is being able to encounter life, which includes personal trials and loss, without succumbing to bitterness and resentment. We also need to realize that the appropriate initial reaction to transitions of the body (for men or women), like any other important change, includes grief and mourning. Bereavement for the body helps us make the transition to a different perspective on life. It is wrestling with these transitions that eventually reshapes the landscape of our inner and outer worlds. Facing both the real and symbolic meaning of loss as it relates to being a man can make one more aware of the vividness of life; this carries the potential of opening up new vistas of insight, purpose, and yes, even feeling.

There is the potential to learn powerful new lessons, lessons rightfully claimed as wisdom. Sometimes the truth we learn comes in the form of being more aware of others' suffering because we have come to know our own. Sometimes it is about forgiveness, as we learn that understanding others more fully often leads to the possibility of compassion, even for those who've left marks upon our hearts. Other times it is about reprioritizing our lives and loving people, not things. Sometimes it can be learning about the sweetness of life only in the last days of living. One may find as many redemptive truths in this personal desert as there are paths to it. These truths reorient us toward our new identities as wiser, gentler people.

I suppose the moral of the story is that the body can break, but that doesn't mean the masculine spirit has to as well. As a partner, family member, or friend, you may have to help in the transition that occurs with normal aging or when the body changes ahead of schedule. Men can find meaning in this process, and it helps by staying hooked to a viable notion of what it means to be a man. For some this will certainly involve a reshuffling of what being a man means. This includes challenging the commandments and the Man Checklist, which for many should have been jettisoned long ago.

In our culture, the media contributes to the skewed view of aging. Television and product marketing places a special emphasis on the rewards of youth culture, and this, in turn, affects how manhood is defined, presented, and packaged. One may wonder if it is possible to retain a feasible notion of masculinity with gray hair, or if you can be a successful middle-aged man without a stockpile of Viagra. Sometimes we lose sight of the fact that an authentic notion of being a man is far more pliable and complex than the two-dimensional definitions we are often pitched. Most of the media front-runners display a very narrow view of what it means to be a man.

In Sophocles' ancient Greek play *Oedipus Rex*, the Sphinx brings a curse to the city of Thebes. It sits outsides the town asking a mysterious riddle, devouring those who answer incorrectly. The Sphinx asks, "What walks on four legs in the morning, two legs at noon, and three legs in the evening?" The answer is "man." In his youth he crawls, in his prime he walks, and in old age, he uses a cane. For modern man, to not know that manhood has different seasons, and with it differing acceptable notions of masculinity, will lead to a modern version of being devoured by the Sphinx.

## New Country for Wise Old Men

Many of the themes discussed in this chapter are visible in the recent Academy Award–winning movie *No Country for Old Men*. Even the title suggests a rather unfriendly reception for men who find themselves at life's transition point, unable to fulfill the roles of protector, provider, and pro-genitor (the Three Ps). In the movie, Tommy Lee Jones plays aging Sheriff Ed Tom Bell, who presides over a West Texas border town, feeling weary and out of sorts trying to combat the crimes of the day. Criminals seem far more ruthless and violent than ever before, and he wonders if there is any-thing he can do to effectively fight them. He goes to consult his Uncle Ellis, a former lawman. We discover that Sheriff Bell's father was killed in the line of duty, and Uncle Ellis, who now sits in a wheelchair, was nearly fatally wounded under similar circumstances.

Uncle Ellis tells his nephew that the region has always been violent, hearkening back to the time of settlers who had fierce encounters with the indigenous people of the area. He shares a story about a lawman who was dragged off his porch one evening and brutally beaten and killed. He accuses Bell of "vanity" in thinking that he could personally make a difference, citing the only two viable ways to end his career: dead (or maimed), or walking away now before it is too late. Shortly afterward, Sheriff Bell retires.

This scene is powerful, but for the wrong reasons. It resonates with the Three Ps and Uncle Ellis's Man Checklist's assumption that physical prowess is the only thing a male has to offer. In Uncle Ellis's view, when those days are over, so is the chance for a viable sense of masculinity. Uncle Ellis lives alone in a run-down cabin; clutter and refuse are everywhere. The coffee on his stove is a week or more old. This is not a man living out his last days in a simple way, but rather a reflection of personal decay. This man is waiting to die, feeling his usefulness has more than run its course. There is not a next step in life's journey for Uncle Ellis, and yet there could be one.

In many mythic tales and stories about heroes, there is the appearance of a wise man character. He possesses special wisdom others eagerly wish to access. Certainly, his days of physical prowess are behind him. However, the wise man's contribution is an integral one, without which the hero could not accomplish his mission. He comes by his special knowledge based in part on having the long view of life; however, this in itself does not guarantee wisdom. He derives understanding from reflection, study, and observation of his own life and those around him. There is also a willingness to share his perceptions with others. The wise man sees real purpose in his later years, and in many cases, those feelings are heightened by the ensuing mystery of death. Because of this, life becomes richer, deeper, and more precious, like vintage wine.

In the movie No Country for Old Men, Uncle Ellis has the potential to be this type of wise man for his nephew but falls short. He could say to Sheriff Bell that a man is more than his youthful pursuits, that there is a time to transition and pass on some duties to younger men, and that the next phase of life can be rewarding as well. He could suggest that Sheriff Bell get involved in training younger officers or consulting on cases. As we see in the movie, youth does not guarantee success in law enforcement, and

Officer Bell has an uncanny sense of observation and instinct that has been honed over the years. These would be valuable tools to pass on to the next generation of officers. But Uncle Ellis cannot say these words of wisdom, because he has not embraced the role that lies beyond the Three Ps.

In comparison, the book *Tuesdays with Morrie* chronicles the fulfilled wise man theme in contemporary society. Mitch Albom rekindles a friendship with his old college professor, twenty years postgraduation. Morrie shares years of wisdom each Tuesday with his life pupil. They talk of love, family, ambition, spirituality, life, and even death, just a few months before the wise man himself passes on. In one conversation, after assessing the state of his own body, Morrie concludes it would not be fair to judge him by his chronological age, because various parts of him feel younger.

This is an important point to consider alongside striving for the Three Ps. Even when men are not able to fulfill the Three Ps like they once did, some men can still find solace in fulfilling an approximation of them. For instance, a financial planning magazine recently featured a picture of a retirement-age man who was grinning from ear to ear. The caption announced that he had just discovered a way to help finance his grandchildren's college education. While not everyone will be in the place to accomplish such a feat, or those like it in terms of the Three Ps, they can still make a contribution to the welfare of others in various ways.

The take-home message is this—there needs to be a new country for wise old men. Wisdom can be siphoned from life's many occurrences, some of which can involve the fulfillment of the Three Ps when done in a responsible and mature way; others may transcend the initial set of personal or cultural rules for being a man when there is a skewed legacy. Still others may discover new ways to define being masculine, ones not solely dependent on the body's status or condition.

Perhaps the status of being a man is intangible, something individually derived from a life well lived, where a man is comfortable in his own skin and connected to those he loves. Aging may afford some men the freedom to become the man they really are, not the one they have often been told to be.

A next phase of mature masculinity can be a reality. It is important to know men that have successfully gone before on these journeys and are able and willing to share what lies ahead. They are more than scribes, chronicling "ancient history"; they can also provide connection, guidance, and valuable emotional support for others. The role of an "elder" should be as it is in Native American tribes: a position of honor and respect. Men must start training for this role now in their younger days, or at least become aware that making that transition someday is not something to be feared. After all, while chronological age can be a factor in reconsidering a personal checklist and the fulfillment of the Three Ps, life can throw you a curve, resulting in a shift sooner than expected.

# Conclusion

The body is a playing field on which a male potentially sorts out his notion of being a man. The highlight film includes experiences as diverse as joys, conflicts, and transitions. Initially, changes in the corporeal being represent the tangible confirmation of having arrived in terms of adult privileges. The Three Ps, the pillars upon which many set the foundation of manhood, guides much of this. Even when the introduction to manhood accompanies fanfare and celebration, men learn that with adult privileges come adult responsibilities. There is a real pressure to succeed at the manly tasks set before you, leading to a rise in rank, prestige, and power, but all the while, you must never let anyone see you sweat. One should accomplish all Herculean tasks with an effortless attitude of "Aw shucks, did I do that?"

Following the traditional notions of masculinity may teach men their bodies are simultaneously a tool for getting what they want in the Darwinian competition of limited social goods but also as a way to hide things labeled as unmanly or taboo. The response by some men is to become more masculine in literal or symbolic ways. This provides a psychological armor to encase male insecurities. But there are moments when the body seems to betray us, either through aging or when the bulletproof vest fails. This allows the normal questions regarding issues of work and love to seep in but also the dysfunctional messages society has established about masculinity. After all, longstanding uncertainties or conflicts do not disappear with the advent of facial hair or muscles.

While men may experience moments of "full exposure" as failures, such occurrences actually can be opportunities that lead to a more authentic and potentially lasting notion of what it means to be a man. This definition is not bound to the temporal functioning of the body, but rather establishes a more permanent place in the psychological realm. Even with this switch, however, men are still required to "workout." The ultimate rewards are not acquiring a six-pack or some really big guns but beefing up in more intangible ways. This type of exercise regime asks participates to delve into areas of mental and emotional vulnerability, so in the end, they become stronger than once thought possible.

# CHAPTER CUES

1. Masculinity is often defined by the ability to achieve three major roles: protector, provider, and progenitor (the Three Ps).

2. There is a personal Man Checklist based on the Three Ps that emphasizes tangible markers of masculinity, each of which centers on the development of the body and its prowess.

3. A skewed rite-of-passage mentality is often applied to masculinity where men are taught to master their bodies by not feeling physical sensations or emotions.

4. The Man Checklist is confusing and limiting because it emphasizes only a young man's notion of masculinity, yet it governs men across the life span.

5. Men can relate to their bodies: (1) in accordance with the commandments, that bigger is better, affording special considerations and opportunities, (2) as a means to compensate for deeper insecurities, and (3) as an emotional vent to discharge conflicted but unacknowledged emotions.

6. The mind/body connection is important for men. Sometimes their emotional conflicts are confused with body sensations like chest pain, upset stomach, headaches, and so on.

7. The (re)establishment of emotional awareness can come through being in touch with bodily sensations and their accompanying feelings.

8. With aging, men may go through a period of adjustment when their bodies begin to change or fail; personal meaning can be found in these transitions.

9. A viable notion of masculinity can be seen across the life span; too often, the media portrays the only acceptable way to be a man is based on youth culture.

10. There needs to be a new country for wise old men; age can afford a new sense of masculinity not based solely on the Three Ps.

PART II

# THE
# GROWING-UP
# YEARS

# 5

# Peter Pan Doesn't Live Here Anymore

Understanding the secret lives of men requires a deep look into the male psyche, and this involves comprehending some of the fantasies that swirl around in men's heads. The word *fantasy* sometimes throws people off because it is too commonly associated with sexuality. When we use the word fantasy in this chapter, we are referring more to daydreams, hopes, or wishes that a little boy has. They are probably not based in objective reality, nor will many of them ever come to pass. As a boy, these hopes or dreams are age-appropriate, but for various reasons, some men don't outgrow them when they become adults.

Boyhood fantasies appear in many different forms. For instance, little boys may fantasize about helping win the Super Bowl by conjuring up last-minute heroics in which they help some of their favorite sports heroes. They fantasize about stepping into a sports scenario and coming up big: "Okay, sports fans, only ten seconds left on the clock; the Pittsburgh Steelers are down by five. It looks like they're going to need a miracle to pull this one off. With the starting quarterback injured, the Steelers are going to their rookie, Chris. Who is this kid coming out of nowhere? They hike the ball. The blitz is on. Chris sidesteps a linebacker, and another. My God, look at that kid's moves! He scrambles to his left . . . back to his right . . .

caught by a linebacker. He is being pulled down. Ouch, that's going to leave a mark! But wait, he still makes the throw! That's a fifty-yard pass right into the hands of his favorite receiver. Chris has won the game! Chris has won the game!"

The thing to appreciate is that this type of elaborate fantasy doesn't happen while a boy is suited up in sports gear in some covered dome arena. It happens in the front yard of his parents' house. Astroturf is easily replaced by chopped-up grass; lawn ornaments and shrubs turn into players from the opposing team that give chase and are to be avoided. A lone garbage can turns into his favorite sports hero who he somehow miraculously throws the ball to, as shrubs—I mean linebackers—pull him down to the weedy St. Augustine turf. And if he doesn't complete the pass squarely into the garbage can, then he has to replay the whole thing again and again until his favorite receiver catches the ball. When his mom says it's time to come inside for supper, the little boy's reply is "Ten more minutes!" I mean, doesn't Mom know the fate of the entire season—no wait, the entire sports franchise—depends on this pass?

Other boyhood fantasies connect more with how the world should be "fair" and people should get what they deserve, good or bad: "That person is mean; why should they get chosen before me?" Some fantasies involve not wanting to share their things or those they love with others ("That's mine, mine, mine, until I don't want it anymore, but I always have the right to reclaim it when I do"), or remembering how it was as a child to bask in the glory of a loving but biased parent. Everything the boy did was golden; even drawings of stick-figure people and dogs got put on the refrigerator, the ultimate place of honor: "I bet even Leonardo da Vinci got his start on a green Kenmore upright as well." These fantasies are age-appropriate for a boy, but when they linger too long into adulthood, they can cause trouble.

All of these fantasies originate in the emotionally primitive world of boyhood. This is the time frame before a manly persona is created; it is raw, sometimes intense, and not always pretty, but it is always authentic. In the emotional realm of a boy, this authenticity allows for an unfiltered experience of the world. In the best moments, it can lead to experiences that feel magical, bordering on the sublime. Those types of encounters are pure octane; they could be harnessed as an alternative fuel source. On occasion, boyhood fantasies can be shared with friends down the street. When this occurs, it becomes the stuff that is etched into the minds of kids for the rest of their lives. While kids think their fantasies go unnoticed by their parents, those who sneak a peek, or even better yet, join in, are transported back in time to the joy they once experienced themselves.

Sadly, some men become separated from the joy of boyhood fantasy as they "grow up." It seems incompatible for some that one can be a man and still stay in touch with boyhood's important essence. After all, when you become a man, you put away childish things, right? But life as a man without a connection to this spirit makes the world seem rather drab, and this can have varying detrimental effects. A man can turn into a type of robot who punches the clock every morning at work and then goes through the motions until quitting time. He may perform the things required of him, but not really take joy in what he does.

A man may lose the spontaneity he once had in his romantic relationship. Playtime with the kids lacks the imagination he once had himself. Then one day he looks up, and he's in his midfifties, having an annual health exam, with his doctor asking, "Are you depressed?" "Of course not, how can I be depressed? I have been this way all of my adult life." The prospect of this kind of life can seem like a punishment conjured up by mythological gods.

The other side of this coin is that some men may have specific areas in their lives where the joy of being a boy is present, but it has transmuted into some twisted thing. Yes, they still have that boyish quality that many romantic partners find irresistible—at first. They can charm others with their impish authenticity and vulnerability. As long as nothing is asked of them in terms of commitment or responsibility, they are fun to be with. The problem, however, is that they have never really grown up. Regarding his romantic relationships, he may think along these lines: "Yeah, she is nice enough alright; I think I do love her, and maybe there could even be a future for us. But right now I just want to concentrate on my music." What he fails to appreciate is that he is well beyond thirty years old, still lives in the basement of his mom's house, and the garage band that he plays in can only book gigs at the coffee shop where his drummer works. His woman is the best thing to come along in his life in quite some time, but the prospect of settling down seems too cumbersome, and let's face it, kind of scary.

Problems with growing up also find their way into work and career areas. A man may move from one job to the next because he feels unappreciated: "Doesn't my boss know that I once helped win the Super Bowl on the front lawn of my parents' house?! Well, that's not something you put on your résumé, but the potential is there for me to do the same thing for this company." And who knows, maybe he could make big contributions for his employer if he would only come to work on a regular basis and not blame "the man" for keeping him down.

Neither one of the above-mentioned alternatives seems very satisfying. One man lives a joyless life, and the other never really grows up. Yet many men feel they need to choose one of these two paths. In this chapter, we look at what I refer to as the Peter Pan Man: those men who have not matured in certain areas of their lives and still hold on to boyhood fantasies that need to be given up. In the next chapter, we look at Lost Boys: men who lose touch with too much of the magic of boyhood and now have joyless lives.

As a romantic partner, there may be aspects of one of these types that you recognize. If your partner is someone who never grew up, you may wonder if his attitudes about work or love are healthy or normal. In the wee hours of the night, you may lie awake and worry about his ability to be a provider, partner, or parent in the long haul. On the other hand, if you recognize that your partner is living in a joyless world, it will give you insight into how this came to be and, ultimately, if there is anything that can be done about it. I will provide warning signs and remedies for when these conditions are potential job or relationship killers, so look for the *Wake-up Calls* and *Toolbox Tips* in each chapter.

# Peter Pan

I think that J. M. Barrie's classic tale *Peter Pan* should be required reading for anyone trying to understand men better. A quick overview of the
story may be helpful, because we will refer to it throughout the next two
chapters. Peter Pan appears at the second-story window of the home of
Wendy and her two brothers. Peter and Wendy, at first glance, seem to be
about the same age. Both are still prepubescent children. Wendy's brothers
are younger still. Peter flies into the window accompanied by Tinker Bell,
the fairy, and after charming Wendy and her two brothers, Peter convinces
them to fly off to Neverland with him. Peter gives the excuse that there are
boys back in Neverland who are in need of a mother's care (himself
included), and Wendy seems like a good candidate for the job. She can tell
stories and has shown herself to be resourceful by sewing Peter's wayward
shadow onto his foot.

During their time in Neverland, they all have wondrous adventures with
Peter as the captain and tour guide of all that is fun. This includes seeing
giant crocodiles and mermaids, fighting with Indians, and defeating the evil
Captain Hook, the pirate who swears vengeance upon Peter for cutting off
his hand and leaving him with an iron hook. Peter Pan and Wendy become
make-believe mother and father of all the other boys in very innocent ways
as the boys look to her for nurturance and Peter for adventure. Then the
whole thing begins to unravel. Wendy asks Peter about his feelings for her,
and he replies that it is all make-believe, not understanding there is more
to a grown-up relationship than the world of pretend. Making matters
worse, Wendy and her brothers begin to forget their real lives before coming to Neverland, including their parents' names and what they look like.
Wendy, growing alarmed about the traps of Neverland, tells Peter she is
leaving, along with her brothers, and taking the other boys, too.

Peter sees them back home where there is a joyful celebration for everyone except him and Wendy. Peter realizes that if he stays in Wendy's world,
they will make him grow up, go to school, and eventually work at an office.

Wendy tells Peter she likes the idea of him being a mature man with a beard, but Peter will have none of this. He promises to fetch Wendy once a year to help him with the spring-cleaning of his house in Neverland. Due to the time difference between Neverland and the real world, or perhaps because of Peter Pan's self-absorption, his visits are rare.

When he does return on one occasion, Wendy has become a wife and mother. When she asks him about the happenings of Neverland as she knew it—Captain Hook, pirates, and mermaids—he does not remember them; even Tinker Bell, the fairy who drank poison to save Peter's life, is lost to his recollection. Others have come and gone and been replaced in his attention and memory. Since Wendy has grown up and is no longer a real candidate for Neverland, Peter takes Wendy's daughter in her place. We are told that, when she grows up, he will take her daughter, and so on, with this cycle continuing forever.

While I have condensed much of the story, the source of real tension is if Peter Pan will stay a boy or grow up, and how this has an impact upon his ability to experience mature life beyond that of the make-believe world in which he lives. These same questions could be posed about the modern-day equivalent: the Peter Pan Man. Will he grow up and be able to assume a job beyond that of fighting make-believe pirates? Will he come to understand mature love with all its complexities, responsibilities, and rewards? Before we answer those questions, let's briefly talk about how the Peter Pan Man ended up this way in the first place.

## What Makes a Peter Pan Man

A Peter Pan Man is created under one or more of the following circumstances: (1) he has not been encouraged to really grow up in particular areas of his life, (2) the methods used to help him grow up were too harsh, or (3) he has experienced emotional trauma that leads to emotional arrest. In either case, the now grown-up man has parts of himself that are still emotionally stuck at a much younger age.

Ultimately, each of these three paths relates to the commandments by way of the man-making blueprint that has enjoyed prominence for more than 100 years. It has mostly gone unchallenged as the tried and true method until just recently. The blueprint for how to change a boy into a man is based on one of Freud's most influential works, *Three Theories of Sexuality*. Later, psychoanalyst Ralph Greenson added to this, forming a two-pronged man-making strategy. To quickly summarize: Step 1 involves severing ties with Mom and all she represents; you may remember the earlier discussion about the fear of the feminine, which is very applicable here. According to the man-making theory, if the boy does not leave the world of the feminine behind, his sense of masculinity is in danger of being thwarted. Step 2 involves finding a father figure/male role model for the boy to imitate; in essence, the older male teaches the boy how to become a man.

This whole plan may seem very familiar as it is encountered repeatedly in TV dramas and books of all kinds. It causes moms (including single moms) a great deal of anxiety. They get the message to not only get out of the way (because they may corrupt their son's sense of masculinity), but at the same time to find a male role model for the boy to emulate.

Recent research has called this whole boy-to-man process into question. Psychologists have suggested that what is being asked of the boy in this process can actually be very harmful. This includes the whole notion of clearly severing a connection with his mom. While Freud suggested this process should happen around five years of age, Greenson argued that it should happen even earlier, when the boy is around two. In theory, the boy should begin moving toward total self-sufficiency and rid himself of anything feminine in the process. This has been interpreted as including the innate emotional and relational qualities like tenderness, vulnerability, and need for others.

While being the accepted model for manhood-making for some time, clinicians and researchers have recently stated this "normal process" is anything but, and that it can cause psychological and emotional trauma. It can lead to "relational dread," which is feeling as though connecting with another is actually a violation of the deepest core of masculine values. It can also foster anger toward those who have "abandoned" him (i.e., Mom) as well as devaluing their contribution to his emotional development—"Don't need that stinky, girly stuff like emotions anyway." What this process does is leave a mark, creating an incomplete and potentially wounded person. Beginning at a young age, this training can interrupt a man's other areas of human development, like being in tune with bodily sensations and emotions.

Growing up is an important endeavor; it cannot happen if someone is cut off at the knees or asked to disavow a part of who they are as a human being. One way to think about it is to imagine what would happen if you stopped feeding a young boy essential vitamins and food; his physical growth would actually be stunted. He would fail to continue along the normal path of physically developing into a strong boy. He may be shorter than normal, have brittle bones, and be more susceptible to disease. Essentially, some boys are left with the emotional equivalent of this type of undernourishment, which can affect them for the rest of their lives. We withhold the essential emotional nutrients found in the recommended daily allowance of care because we are still buying into an outdated blueprint for how boys are supposed to become men. The sad truth is that this blueprint has resulted in emotionally stunted men.

Also, there is the psychological impact on the boy when the older male role model who is supposed to shape his sense of masculinity is either physically or emotionally absent and carries his own wounds about being a man. The boy may make a leap of faith, trusting that breaking ties with Mom and the feminine is in his best interests (i.e., the grown-up thing to do) only to be shortchanged by a father figure who cannot supply any real guidance or connection. The boy may fill the vacuum with more anger, apathy, or an array of psychological defenses that only prolongs his psychological arrest.

One potential reaction to the trauma of the man-making blueprint is the creation of a Peter Pan Man, one who flies away from the fear of the feminine, old wounds created from feeling abandoned, and anything resembling the adult world. After pairing all the man-making training with the notion that growing up is actually good for you, one can imagine that further encouragement along this line doesn't carry a lot of water. "If that is what it means to be a grown-up, you can keep it!"

Of course, this type of response will affect his ability to work or love in the long run. Some men show they are stuck in Neverland by still carrying the fear and anxiety of the treatment they experienced as a boy well into adulthood; they are timid and fearful men who are unable to do well in the grown-up world. Sometimes they may feel like powerless little boys surrounded by grown-ups. Other men respond like Peter Pan and try to fly high above the troubles they have experienced by entering into a permanent type of make-believe. It is this way of responding to the demands of growing up that will occupy our time in this chapter.

## ▶ Toolbox Tip: What Is Good Nurturing Anyway?

Given that the man-making blueprint frowns on nurturing, it may be beneficial to discuss what it can be in the healthiest sense. Contrary to what some may believe, nurturing is not something that belongs exclusively to the world of women. Nurturing: it does a psyche good. Nurturing involves finding the right balance of support and challenge. It includes all the aspects that normally come to mind, like love, warmth, and valuing someone. But it also pertains to being firm in difficult situations when you know it is best for someone, supplying corrective feedback in a caring way, and allowing someone to be his or her own person. Both genders are capable of supplying this type of nurturing: moms, dads, brothers, sisters, girlfriends, boyfriends, partners, best friends, husbands, and wives.

One of the most important points to understand is that nurturing, in the sense in which we are defining it, means giving the right balance of support and challenge, which is not a corrupting force to masculinity. Instead, it is what will allow an individual to brave the difficulties of growing up male and help him to come through it a whole person, ready to assume the adult responsibilities of love and work. Robbing boys of this type of nurturing leaves them ill prepared for what lies ahead in the adult world. The old notion that toughening up a boy is the same as depriving him of care does nothing but hobble him. More about the specifics of nurturing will be given in Chapter 11, which is about "guardians," the special people in a man's life who assume this role.

# Peter Pan Men in Adult Life

Initially, the Peter Pan Man is not always easily spotted. His personality can be disarming and can lure a potential romantic interest into thinking he or she has found Mr. Right. A Peter Pan Man knows how to have fun, and his lust for life can be intoxicating to those around them. He can also win you over with boyish flashes of vulnerability, which can entice you into a protective mothering role. You may never feel as alive as you do when you're with a Peter Pan Man. This has a lot to do with one of his endearing qualities—his level of authenticity. Authenticity means truly being one's self. Most of us know what that feels like, and we are reminded of it when we see little kids at play. There are no fronts; their emotions are real, raw, and intense. So, what's so wrong with being authentic? Nothing—if we know how to cultivate and express it in appropriate ways.

One time I was giving a presentation about boys and authenticity, stressing its importance in living a healthy life. One of the audience members raised a very important question. She worked with troubled adolescents in a group home, and she said if she allowed those boys to really be *authentic*, they would be at one another's throats. It is true for all of us that being authentic can sometimes mean showing parts of ourselves that are authentically hurt, broken, demanding, or angry. This situation is intensified when, like those boys in the group home, important aspects of nurturing were chronically absent growing up. In those cases, people not only feel the burden of having missed out on what was needed, but they are prone to have less restraint about showing their troubles in explosions of hurt or anger. It takes a certain level of emotional development not to act out in destructive ways when feeling intense emotions, and to achieve this status, you have to receive at least a minimal amount of care.

A Peter Pan Man can share a similar dilemma with the group home boys—he also missed out on important emotional nurturing and has trouble controlling his emotions when he feels let down. This can result in him being thin-skinned, prone to show his hurt or damaged parts in very edgy ways. In the grown-up world of work and love, that approach can become very destructive. In growing up, there is a certain tension between being authentic and knowing how to package those feelings, thoughts, and behaviors in suitable ways. The Peter Pan Man would say that being a grown-up is too stifling. He thinks he should just be able to do what feels good without any limits or restraint. He might even accuse you of being a boring adult when you suggest to him that not every disappointed emotion has to be acted on.

There are many other ways his difficulty with tolerating frustration shows itself. For instance, Peter Pans have a tendency to replace people in their lives very quickly. If you won't "play with them," they will go off and find someone who will. Imagine a little boy working through the kids on the playground, staying with each one as long as he is entertained, and then moving on when the fun is over. That is the playground mentality of a Peter Pan Man. Their initial charm can open some doors in meeting others, but their limited emotional resources don't allow them to handle frustration or disappointment well.

Since dealing with letdowns is a necessary skill in making lasting connections, the end results are often a series of intense but short relationships. Just last week, he may have given you the impression that you are special to him. After all, someone who knows how to fly has picked you for his partner. But just like in the story, when Wendy asks Peter Pan how he really feels about her, his response may be to say, in so many words, "What are you talking about? This is all make-believe." It is fun to pretend you are grown-ups in love, but just like the original Peter Pan, yours may not really understand or have the emotional skills to go beyond make-believe.

Peter Pans of the world can be disappointing, and at times, hurtful, especially if seen as, or expected to be more than, what they are: adult men with the emotional functioning of a boy. They are a mixed bag of charm, vulnerability, self-absorption, and paralyzing fear. If the man you love is a full-blown Peter Pan, the odds are against his being ready for the responsibilities of the adult world, specifically, work and love. The bottom line is that being married to a Peter Pan Man, and to an even greater extent having a family together, would have its significant challenges. For a short time, he would be a lot of fun. There are times when his boyish charm is endearing, but he's not the kind of man you can build a future with.

## WAKE-UP CALL:
### How to Identify a Peter Pan Man

1. You hear too often that commitment is an overblown concept.
2. In his life, people are easily replaced.
3. He has a history of feeling like jobs or relationships are a constant infringement upon his freedom.
4. He has a blank stare when asked what he thinks being in a mature relationship really means.
5. He has lived off of his boyish charm at work or in relationships while really making no substantial contributions.
6. He pulls for a maternal reaction from you that lets him off the hook from adult responsibilities, like keeping a job or doing the needed work in a relationship.

## WAKE-UP CALL:
### Living in Neverland Can Become Disorienting

If you find yourself in the role of Wendy with your Peter Pan Man, keep in mind that being in Neverland too long can become disorienting. Remember, in the original Peter Pan story, Wendy, along with her brothers, began losing touch with the real world. Such is the power of being in Neverland; it causes people to question those things they knew for certain before they entered that magical realm.

The modern equivalent of this Wendy dilemma is when you begin to normalize situations that are not at all normal: for instance, you are working three jobs, and your Peter Pan Man is unemployed but making significant strides as an online poker player. Or, he says that infidelity is a normal part of most couples' troubles, and that just because he has a history of leaving his other romantic partners, surely that doesn't apply to you.

If you find yourself forgetting the rules and responsibilities that govern what normal life is like, you may need to revisit old familiar things or people that provide a sense of grounding. Remember, Wendy's solution was to head back home. Sometimes finding a space that feels that way can help you clarify the direction you're heading in and help you decide if you want to really go there. Create a temporary Peter Pan Man–free zone where you can go to think and sort things out.

# Breaking the Neverland Barrier

If you are committed to being with your Peter Pan Man, there are some things he, and consequently you, are up against in terms of his growing up. There are a number of things he must implement before he can transition into the adult world. This involves breaking the Neverland barrier that keeps him insulated in a boylike mentality.

Think of the Neverland barrier as an imaginary wall that separates the world of a boy from that of a man. (Girls also have their own version of a Neverland barrier that needs to be crossed in order to become a woman, but Peter Pan Man will be our focus here.) In the best of all situations, a boy crosses the Neverland barrier when he is adequately prepared to do so, and while it may be a bit of a stretch in terms of effort, the journey opens a whole new world to him. He sees people, relationships, and difficult situations with new eyes. He knows what it means to be loyal and steadfast, how to hold the line in tough times, as well as realizing when it is time to soften and be compassionate to himself and those he loves. He is a go-to guy. You trust him with your life. Because of that trust, real intimacy is possible; but there is also something more—it stokes the flames of romance in the bedroom. A mature man can be an attentive and satisfying lover. In the very best situation, a grown man retains some of the charm and authenticity from youth because he is comfortable in his own skin. Others feel drawn to him because of that. He can honestly be called a good man.

The hard thing is that the Peter Pan Man does not realize a healthy transformation is possible; he has not seen what lies on the other side of the Neverland barrier. Instead, he thinks he has it good where he is, and there is no real reason to move on. The Peter Pan Man does not realize that growing up adds a whole new dimension to life. Let's look at the challenges a Peter Pan Man must understand and put into effect if he is to cross the Neverland barrier and become a grown man: (1) A Peter Pan Man must realize that growing up is not synonymous with death or personal oblivion; (2) The escape from Neverland is about committing to the steady day-today effort involved in work and love; and (3) Everyday responsibilities can bring joy into life.

*Challenge No. 1*: A Peter Pan Man must realize that growing up is not synonymous with death or personal oblivion. This is easier said than done. The main reason he holds to this belief is that he has not successfully crossed the threshold of boyhood mentality in any significant area of his life. The thought of heading out into such an unknown journey is terrifying. He fears he would not endure such an expedition and live to tell about it.

Jungian analyst Marie Louise von Franz discussed one of the deeper psychological reasons the Peter Pan Man balks at crossing the Neverland barrier. She asserted that, whether it relates to his commitment to work or love, it is fear which holds a Peter Pan Man back—fear that he will lose himself if he takes one step too many in the direction of adulthood. There is always that fork in the road when approaching the Neverland barrier; having already come so far, should he go a little farther? The Peter Pan Man weighs the potential consequences of that next step and what it may cost him. This is where fear can consume him. He thinks if he goes one step too far—buys the minivan instead of the sports car, decides he really will dig in to his new job in earnest, or throws away his little black book and commits to one person—it is a small distance to personal oblivion. He worries that a stranger will be looking back at him when he looks in the mirror.

People are resistant to change, even if they know it is for the best, because they are fearful of the unknown. They would rather stick with what's familiar, even if it costs them friends, jobs, and partners. The Peter Pan Man will begin looking for greener pastures where growing up will not be necessary. When he has charted this course, he will fly away.

In those crucial moments, when he is standing on the edge and his next decision will either lead to a mature change for the better or continue the cycle of fear and self-destruction, he may clearly see what truly frightens him. If you can take hold of his wings before he flies off and ask him in your kindest "Wendy" voice what he is afraid of, he may look at you to see if you really want to know. He is sizing you up to see if you are sturdy enough to hear his deepest fears. You nod. He says, "I am afraid I will turn into [insert the name of the person he fears becoming]." No doubt there is a picture in his mind of a *corrupted* adult, someone who, by Peter Pan standards, has a joyless existence. You may hear the story of an overachieving father who worked himself into an early grave, or a mother who loved so deeply it broke her heart when her partner left. He may say he would rather die than be like them.

Another question that may be worth asking the Peter Pan Man is, "What are you afraid of experiencing *again?*" Remember, some Peter Pan Men employ their flying technique to distance themselves from the overwhelming pain of the past. To stand still, firmly rooted, is to run the risk of feeling those things all over again. The Peter Pan Man approach is to keep stirring, never really settling into jobs or relationships; there is less chance of being hurt if you never really get too close to others or show your own vulnerability. In the movie *Magnolia*, Tom Cruise does a wonderful job of portraying one of these wounded Peter Pan Men. When his father abandoned the family at an early age, he was left as a young boy to tend to his dying mother. This, of course, is beyond what little boys are meant to do—it leaves a mark. It is too painful for him to experience those memories. His way of protecting himself against their painful recollection is to fly above them, in an angry, distant way.

Some Peter Pan Men *fly*, not because they want to, but because they have to. To land is to come into contact with old hurts from the past. The author of the Peter Pan story, J. M. Barrie, knew this as well. He had a very difficult childhood, filled with pain and the tragic death of his brother. His response was to never grow up by adult standards; instead, he stayed close to the world of make-believe. When he wrote about Peter Pan, chances are he had an insider's view of what Neverland was really like.

These insights into the world of the Peter Pan Man can soften partners' and friends' reactions to the question, "Why the hell won't he just grow up?!" It has to be understood that growing up can be scary in the best of situations, and for some men, that fear becomes even more intensified because it means facing the emotional damage of the past. Sometimes, breaking the Neverland barrier involves dealing with the lingering pain from long ago in an honest way. Doing this changes a person. It does not necessarily have to change the flavor of his personality, as some people fear; it just makes him a higher-functioning version of his old self. The Peter Pan Man does not have to lose a zest for life; he just needs to learn how to function better in the adult world. Later in this book, there are two chapters devoted to helping all men, including Peter Pans, make peace with the legacy of a painful past. If the Peter Pan Man breaches the barrier in this process, he makes room for the possibility that other areas may also follow.

*Challenge No. 2: The escape from Neverland is about committing to the steady day-to-day effort involved in work and love.* The response by the Peter Pan Man to this notion is, "I don't want to!" One of the mistakes partners and friends make is expecting him to have a smooth transformation into a grown-up state without any backsliding. This is an unrealistic hope that leads to frustration on everybody's part. To break the Neverland barrier involves a back-and-forth process of adjustment: one step forward and sometimes two back. It has to be worked at until he is finally ready to breach the Neverland barrier.

Sometimes the Peter Pan Man undertakes a new venture in adult living because he really cares about his romantic partner and is trying to be more involved in the relationship. But there is still the question of his default setting of wanting to fly away when things get too complicated or cumbersome. For instance, maybe it is the holidays and your Peter Pan Man is not big on the family thing, but he goes ahead and accompanies you on the visit to see your family anyway because he knows it means a lot to you. You realize it is a bit of a stretch for him, but it makes you feel good inside that he is making the effort. You see him playing in the backyard with all your brother and sister's kids, and he even seems to be enjoying it! And you begin to think, "Wow, he is really turning the corner. Maybe we could talk about taking that next step, settle in, and even have kids of our own someday!" Then during the drive home he comments, "Yeah, that was something, wasn't it! Could you imagine being tied down like that?!! I would go mad."

Other times, the Peter Pan Man will flirt with the idea of trying something new because it could be entertaining. Even the original Peter Pan liked to pretend he and Wendy were grown-ups in love with a houseful of sons placed in their charge. This could find its way into both areas of love and work: "The idea of starting and keeping a real job could be fun. I get to dress up and carry a briefcase and have a real reason for using my cell phone. Did I tell you I get a business card with my name on it? Pretty cool!" But the real test comes, as Marie Louise von Franz suggested, on those rainy Monday mornings or sunny Friday afternoons when work is the last place he wants to be: "Everybody else is out having fun and I am stuck at this lousy job working . . . grumble . . . grumble . . . grumble." The temptation is to call in sick or just blow the whole thing off: "Yeah, the boss said I have been putting in some really serious hours at work lately, so he told me I should just work from home today."

A Peter Pan Man has to approach growing up in small steps. Expecting him to move too quickly will not lead to much success. He will instead begin to pull back and shout things like, "What do you want from me?! I got a job, didn't I? I went to your family's for Christmas; what else is there for me to do?!" The hard thing is that he really is drawing a blank about what comes next; again, he has not successfully crossed the Neverland line that separates boyhood from manhood. Once he has accomplished this task of crossing over in at least one significant area of his life, he has something to draw on in other areas as well. For instance, if he really realizes that going to work every day is essential and the only way to get a paycheck, then chances are he may also eventually learn that the same steadiness is needed for being a partner in a relationship or taking care of children. That is, he learns about the important grown-up qualities of perseverance and loyalty in multiple areas of his life.

*Challenge No. 3: Everyday responsibilities can bring joy into life.* A Peter Pan Man will complain about the everyday duties that go with work and love. In his mind, everything should be exciting all the time. The repetition of everyday life seems potentially loaded with dissatisfaction and boredom.

Have you ever wondered how children can watch the same video twenty times a week? Nauseated parents turn toward the kitchen after putting on the same DVD of Barney, Barbie, Nemo, or whomever, while kids hunker down and are excited about the prospect of seeing their favorite video again. Where does this joy in repetition and seemingly monotonous behavior come from? In part, it has to do with the kids' still-developing brains. When children are exposed to the same material over and over again, they can perceive slight nuances because their little brains are turning on new levels of functioning all the time. What was perceived on one level of depth or complexity one week ago is experienced in a whole new dimension the next. Seeing the same video over and over again helps the child take in all that is there.

As adults, we can relearn this same skill if we move beyond the "been there, done that" mentality. Those who practice living in the moment, truly focused on what they are doing or who they are talking to, even if it seems like the "same old, same old," can discover new levels of joy in what we normally label "mundane." At first blush, this joyless monotony seems to be the nemesis of a Peter Pan Man, but if we look closer, we will see that some of the same creativity he used to make every experience a magical one while he inhabited Neverland transfers to the adult world as well. This is where a former Peter Pan Man really has an advantage. Who else can turn a discarded cardboard box into a fort, ready for his kids to inhabit and defend against the enemy? Who better than a former Peter Pan Man to make a walk in the park or a Friday night at home with a video magical?

## Lingering Too Long in Neverland

While some partners, family members, and friends encounter full-blown Peter Pans like those described above, others notice there are only certain areas where the man in question seems stuck in Neverland; other areas of his life seem fine. Even so, these areas of concern can cause trouble too. To grow up, we have to do some things that are not easy or pleasant. We have to put away some hopes and dreams that will never come to pass, because holding on to them will make life more difficult in the long run. But this does not have to be the same thing as losing boyhood joy, authenticity, or breaking one's spirit. Instead, being able to hold on to boyhood joy makes the transition to the grown-up world easier. It provides psychological padding that will buffer the transition from boy to man.

One of my good friends was going through a difficult potty-training stage with his son. Luke did not want to sit on the training potty; instead, he still preferred to go "poopy" in his pull-ups. He could have chosen a harsh approach like threatening or shaming Luke to get on the potty, but my friend knew this was not how he wanted to handle his son. He realized that Luke's spirit or willfulness would someday blossom into strength, and he did not want to harm it. At the same time, he knew he didn't want his son wearing pull-ups when he was a freshman in college. Something had to be done.

Luke really liked the character Donkey from *Shrek,* so my friend bought a new batch of pull-ups featuring all the *Shrek* characters, including Donkey. Luke tried on the new pulls-ups and looked down at Donkey; he seemed excited but also concerned. My friend said to Luke, "I know they're fun to wear, and I also think you're worried about pooping on Donkey." This made perfect sense to Luke because he didn't want to poopy on Donkey. After all, he was his favorite cartoon character. So he started using the toilet instead. This is a good example of helping a boy adjust to one of the first transitions of growing up. Up to this point Luke could go poopy anywhere and anytime he wanted. Now he had learned that there were appropriate times and places for this. (By the way, Luke's mom made me promise I would mention that he was still well within the age-appropriate phase of pull-ups and not in junior high.)

Psychologically speaking, potty training is really one of the first lessons about authority and rules. This training sets the foundation for other lessons that are learned along the way, like raising your hand in class before you speak or not taking what does not belong to you. If the first experience of authority is a harsh one, aimed at compliance at all costs, including breaking the child's spirit, then authority problems may soon follow. These problems may take the form of railing against authority or caving in too easily to anyone considered an authority.

The importance of being able to let go of certain fantasies like "I can poopy wherever and whenever I want, without regard for others," which can later mutate into "I should have my way all the time," is important. The fun and caring way my friend helped his son allowed for Luke to harness his will to protect Donkey from poopy and, consequently, to learn about limits and rules. But Luke did not have his spirit crushed in the process. He could turn potty training into a fun thing. The more we adopt this approach of harnessing willpower to brave the difficulties of growing up, the better. In the next section, we will discuss some common areas where men get emotionally arrested.

# Some Wishes from Neverland That Must Be Reconciled

There are some plain truths that the Peter Pan Man just simply can't see. They include misperceptions and misconceptions about the realities of how the world really works, including love and relationships, job and career work, and male virility. Though the dilemmas in leaving Neverland are straightforward for the most part, you might notice a softening around the edges on some of these issues if you choose to discuss them with your partner, friend, or family member. Chapter 10, on giving helpful feedback to men, will go into more depth about this. Below are some truths about common areas of life that the Peter Pan Man needs to learn.

## Their Perspective of the World

1. *Life is not fair.* The belief that life is, or at least should be, fair is one of the toughest childhood elements to let go of; however, not doing so can lead to a self-pitying and jaded approach to the world. Some men will hang on to the idea that they were "screwed" growing up: they didn't

get enough of a parent's attention, or their family didn't have money, or they weren't given the advantages others had. These things may all be true, but to use them as a justification for not leaving Neverland can lead to a man's undoing.

2. *If a man missed out on having a male role model, he can still be a real man.* This is a potential offshoot of the "Life is not fair" perspective, but it's about a specific area that male culture emphasizes. Some men struggle with a physically or emotionally absent father. Often men gauge their ability to be a "real man" based on how present their fathers were when they were growing up. Hanging on to this conflict keeps a man from crossing the Neverland barrier. We'll look at this more fully in Chapter 7.

## Work

1. *If a man has not become a sports hero or rock star celebrity by age forty, chances are it won't happen.* Some men will hang on to the boyhood fantasy of becoming a "star" for too long. It hinders them from becoming good providers or from sustaining gainful employment. They will risk it all to pursue a dream that will not happen. Often the dream area has to be turned into a vocation or a hobby. But the danger here is that the same level of intensity or hope for stardom gets transferred to things like coaching Little League, and the children in their charge suffer because of it. Men like these are easily identified because in recreation leagues where the team is made up of five-year-olds they cuss and swear at the kids because, "They don't realize what is at stake." Yes, the dashed dreams of a would-be star now turn into the hope of gaining the "coach of the year" award.

2. *There is no such thing as an ideal work situation; even with a man's dream job there are annoyances.* There is no perfect job. Let me say that again—there is no perfect job. Men who go through ill-advised and frequent job changes because the grass is always greener in

another company end up undermining their careers. They fantasize that their lives will come together when they find the perfect job with no annoyances.

## Expectations for Partners

1. *Being unfaithful is not a legitimate way to act out anger toward a partner or spouse.*

   One thing we learn in junior high romances is that they don't usually last long. Your soul mate one week may be an unknown person to you the next. In early dating relationships, if a boy gets mad at his girlfriend, he might trade her in for someone else or do things to "get even," like date her best friend. If a man doesn't outgrow this kind of behavior, it can lead to a "punish my partner by cheating" approach in adult relationships. This is a relationship disaster.

2. *A man's partner cannot meet all his emotional needs. He has to build meaningful relationships outside of the couple.* This is a tough one for many men. I have heard a fair number of women trying to set up adult "play dates" so their boyfriends or husbands have a "go-to guy" to hang around with. A partner or spouse can be caring and supportive, but they cannot do it all, because that places too much of a burden on the relationship. Some of the emotional needs have to be spread around. It takes a village to feed a man's heart and soul. Plus, if a man expects one person to supply all his emotional requirements, this can lead to an unbalance of power within the romantic relationship. He may feel like "Yes, dear" is the only answer he can ever give, even if that is not how he feels. This unhealthy approach stems from wanting to keep his only viable support system happy at all costs.

3. *There is no such thing as a relationship that won't let you down at times.* Misunderstandings happen in all loving relationships; that is a given. The hard work for some men is moving through misunderstandings so that the hurt is in the past. Or, as Winston Churchill once said, "If you

are going through hell, keep going." Some men need to learn realistic expectations for those they love; at the end of the day, we are all human and have both strengths and limitations.

4. *The areas of communication and emotions are not exclusively the territory of women; men can master those skills as well.* There have been times when I have been working with female psychotherapy clients and they pause and look at me like, "How do you know that about emotions? You're a man!" Men are capable of mastering the realm of emotions.

5. *If he needs to always "be the man," he will soon find himself alone.* While each couple has their own rhythm regarding decision making, if one partner feels like he has to win all the arguments for the sake of winning or be right all the time to show he is in charge, chances are that relationship is doomed.

6. *If a man must defer to his partner on all decisions, he may be in the wrong relationship.* Likewise, if a man feels like he has no decision-making power in the relationship and cannot express himself, he will start acting out in destructive ways. This can take the form of wandering eyes, inappropriate sexual remarks, or even affairs. Sometimes this form of acting out is an indirect expression of anger aimed at the partner or spouse.

## Male Virility

1. *At some point, twenty-one-year-olds won't find him sexually attractive anymore. Instead, they will refer to him as "sir" or "mister."* Every man dreams of maintaining the charm and vitality of youth—that is why hair plugs and Viagra are so popular. But some men don't want to wake up to the realization that aging is a part of life. Men who try to measure their aging manliness by how many young women they can attract are emotionally stuck.

## Expectations for Male Best Friends

1. *While sometimes going to the pub is a needed distraction, drinking too much, too often, with his friends doesn't solve his problems.* Everyone needs a time to decompress, but for some men, they have *special friends* who in reality do little more than drag him into the gutter. Let's not confuse this with blowing off steam or a night out to help him get his bearings back after a hard week's work. Wives and partners can usually identify this special group of friends and know they are a destructive influence that brings their man down instead of lifting him up.

2. *If he really has a best friend, sometimes their conversation needs to move beyond a junior high school level of relating.* I remember a men's support group that I used to run, most of whose members I saw as individual clients first. When I would invite them to join the "men's group" and would tell them we would meet for about an hour and a half, I would sometimes get blank stares about what we would be doing. On one occasion, one man asked me, "Will we be watching TV and drinking beer?" Learning to have a real relationship with others is a skill your man will need to discover, and this is especially true with his best friends.

3. *Even though he may be a grown man, "playtime" is still an important part of a friendship.* Recreation is about re-creating ourselves through connection and play. Sometimes there doesn't have to be too many words passed between men to have a good outing and accomplish this task. So when you ask your partner or spouse, "What did you all talk about when you where playing golf today?" sometimes the honest answer is "nothing."

## Expectations from Sports

1. *Sports teams cannot really provide a sense of family.* A great memoir by Nick Hornby, *Fever Pitch*, illustrates this point very well. During a

rough period growing up, when his parents were divorcing, he found that following his local professional soccer team provided a sense of a dependable family. Unfortunately for him, this became an obsession that followed him into adulthood, impacting his work and family. For instance, he began worrying that special occasions, like weddings and the birth of his children, would fall on game day, and he would have to choose which events to attend. Many men can relate to this type of situation. A sports team can provide what seems like a dependable sense of belonging. The teams' problems, joys, and triumphs become his own, as in a family. But the truth is that sports teams are not family. Your man has to purchase a ticket in order to "visit" them.

2. *He does not have a personal relationship with his sports hero.* If your man has sports memorabilia, like jerseys, signed baseballs, or game day souvenirs, chances are they are associated with his favorite sports player. Owning this stuff gives the impression there is a level of familiarity between him and his idol, like they are old pals. But the truth is, his sports hero doesn't know him from Adam. When was the last time his sports hero called when he was having a bad day?

3. *Prioritize, prioritize, prioritize.* Sports seasons come back each year, but with the important people in his life, he usually only gets one chance.

## Coaxing Someone from Neverland

Having read about some of the different ways a man may get stuck in Neverland, and of the truths he is unable to see, you might feel more compelled than ever to help him. Living in Neverland does not compare to a content existence in the grown-up world. Plus, you no doubt have something at stake here as well, and find yourself irritated, disappointed, or questioning if the relationship can work in the long run. In some situations, professional help may be needed to help sort out why a man's development has become arrested in some areas. Some men have one foot in Neverland and one foot in the real world, and this can be confusing for those who love him.

I think one of the most important things is to be able to adjust the lens through which you view him. He may be a grown man, competent in many areas of his life, but when he bumps up against that area which is still trapped in Neverland, you need to remember that he is revealing a part of himself that is still emotionally a little boy. This does not mean you acquiesce to his demands to remain a child. Rather, to help, you have to approach him the way you would a timid young man. If he has experienced harsh treatment around the area in question, taking a harsh stance now may not only rewound him, it will also get you nowhere in your discussion. All the defenses he has spent years building up will be immediately activated. You run the risk of failing him and of him closing up the secret shoe box to you.

While Chapter 10 offers a more detailed approach on how to deal with these difficult situations, it is enough for right now that you focus on your overall attitude when confronting him about the area in which he is still a Peter Pan Man. Your approach is everything. You may have to put on some emotional armor to prepare yourself for what he has to say. When you are inviting him to reveal who he is, you may not like everything that he says. In hearing these things, you must focus on not shaming him or humiliating him for what seems like a "childish" way of viewing the world, relationships, or the past. I believe that type of treatment becomes one of the deepest types of wounds to a man: feeling like his partner, wife, girlfriend, or daughter does not respect him.

In the next chapter, we will look at the opposite of a Peter Pan Man, the Lost Boy. These Lost Boys are men who crashed through the Neverland barrier and subsequently lost all touch with the magic of boyhood. This joyless existence is reflected in their romantic relationships, careers, and even with their children. We will discuss how to identify them and what can be done to help them.

## ▶ Toolbox Tip: Little Man Picture Technique

One of the techniques you may try involves finding an old picture of him from when he was a boy. You can ask him to tell you the story of the picture, what was going on at the time, what he was like then, and the kinds of things with which he struggled. You are searching for a picture to represent the little man inside of him who is still partially stuck in Neverland. You can carry this picture with you in your purse or place a copy of it on your desk at work—anywhere that will help you connect to that part of him. You will know when the right picture is found. More than likely, similar expressions and gestures will resurface when the little boy gets uncorked. Hold on to this image of him in your mind when you see the same emotional qualities begin to surface now. Let this be the anchoring point for you in these difficult discussions. Imagine doing nothing that would harm that little man. If you can hold on to this place, you may find yourself softening to the annoyance in the moment. This is a first solid step to reclaiming that part of him from the Neverland prison.

## ▶ Toolbox Tip: Roadblocks on the Path to Change

After you have spent some time talking with him about the past, you may find the natural transition is to discuss how this affects him in the present. This could be in the areas of work or love. One of the ways you can help the man who is partially stuck in Neverland is by practicing the following technique: when he begins to talk about what is troubling in the context of how it affects him now, the natural knee-jerk reaction is to say, "Well, change your behavior; what's so hard about that?" For someone who is not emotionally stuck in the area of concern, it may seem straightforward. You may begin to feel impatient or excited and begin to start offering suggestions for how he can change and what he should do. You know you are off course when he begins to say "Yes, but . . ." to every suggestion you offer.

At this point, there is still something blocking his way and keeping him from taking action. Sometimes this can be multiple things. Imagine that you are both on top of a canyon looking down into the valley. Your attitude should be "You don't have to walk down into the canyon right now—but what roadblocks would you encounter on the way?" Questions like this can reveal meaningful things. The roadblocks are often based in fear, whether realistic or not. You may ask something like "Whether it is based in reality or not, what keeps you from going ahead?" Next, prepare yourself for the unexpected, listen, and hold on to the image of the little man in your mind, knowing that the care he missed when he was growing up affected this area of his life. What you are doing is placing healing ointment on this old wound. This will build a deeper sense of trust between you and him.

# Conclusion

Each person (man or woman) has areas in the psyche that need a little fine-tuning. This work often entails dealing with old fantasies that don't belong in the adult world. These fantasies involve skewed expectations of the self, the world, and others. Left in their present unchanged form, such fantasies can cause one to stumble in the areas of work and love. After all, showing up to work in a pirate costume may not get a man the corner office or the girl of his dreams. The hope is that a man may cross over the Neverland barrier in at least one significant area of his life and use that experience as an internal guide for more adult behavior. By doing this, faulty hopes and wishes that stand in the way of more functional relationships and more successful job opportunities are finally laid to rest.

When a man has too many detained areas, he is in danger of becoming a Peter Pan Man: a charming but emotionally arrested fellow with little hope of seeing the other side of the Neverland barrier. That is, unless the right Wendy comes along and compels him to grow up. This Wendy may be a literal person or a symbolic life event, mission, or purpose. It must be something that he commits himself to on a daily basis, something important enough to encourage him to weather the natural ups and downs that come with any situation. This includes sticking to it when things get tough, boring, or even when others outside his window seem to be having all the fun. Following this prescription to fruition means the Peter Pan Man will begin to see the manly stubble of a beard on his once boylike chin. This man must focus on retaining the joy and sense of being alive even as he crosses the Neverland barrier to a more adult world of rewards and responsibilities.

# CHAPTER CUES

1. The Peter Pan Man has never grown up. His being stuck is the result of an emotional arrest that stems from the commandments and the traditional man-making blueprint that has only recently been challenged.

2. Growing up can be tough in the best of situations. The right balance of support and challenge is the model to follow to help raise boys or assist the Peter Pan Man.

3. Peter Pan Men have some serious challenges to face. They may have boyish charm, but they have not learned to be committed to do the day-to-day efforts needed to make work and relationships successful.

4. For the Peter Pan Man to be on his way to grown-up status, he has to successfully cross the Neverland barrier in at least one area of his life.

5. Some otherwise competent men can have parts of themselves that are still stuck in Neverland. This can include areas related to work, love, family, views toward their own children, and sports.

6. As a significant other, parent, or friend, you have to adjust the way you view a grown man in moments of Neverland vulnerability. Try the "little man picture technique" to soften your stance or the "roadblock technique" to help explore possible barriers to change.

# 6

# Lost Boys to Renaissance Men

In the last chapter we discussed the full-blown Peter Pan Man, as well as the man who only has a part of himself stuck in Neverland; both face a similar dilemma when growing up—the loss of innocence. This is not something exclusive to these types of men. All men and women face issues when considering permanently crossing the Neverland barrier into the grown-up world.

A loss of innocence involves seeing and experiencing the world in a much different way than the uncomplicated perspective associated with the formative years. As we mature, we move into a more complex understanding of people, the world, and ourselves. For instance, one moves beyond the simple good and bad dichotomous categorizations of others. Instead, we are forced to integrate more ambiguous pictures of the important people in our lives. Reshuffling our mental and emotional pictures of those we have idealized without reservation in our youth can be a taxing and sometimes painful process.

Likewise, dealing with the "bad people" in our lives requires both the energy and the willingness to see them as flawed human beings whose limitations and subsequent disappointments are often linked to their own legacy of unresolved emotional wounds. Can you justify continuing to abhor someone when you come to understand their damaged personal history? When we start rearranging how we view the important people who have shaped our lives, it will eventually have a domino effect, also impacting how we see ourselves and the world in general.

If we have come to understand others as a complicated mixture of both strengths and limitations, shouldn't we carry out the same exercise with the person in the mirror? This task of self-evaluation invites us to see ourselves in a different light, and at times it can require some real soul-searching. This intricate resorting is not limited to finding new, more mature perspectives of ourselves and others; it also involves our discovery of a fresh way of viewing the world. Is the world fair? Do people get what they deserve? As an adult, is there any way to make things better? These are all complicated issues that clearly belong in the grown-up world, and believe it or not, all this complexity does not have to lead to an overriding sense of mental and emotional clutter.

Sometimes even those firmly ensconced in the grown-up world still have an occasional brush with the forsaken realm of the magical. Usually this occurs when interacting with someone who still fully resides within Neverland, such as a wide-eyed child looking for confirmation that their cherished beliefs are true. It is encountering this level of innocence in its very purest form that momentarily reminds us of simpler times when we cherished an unwavering belief in Santa Claus and the Tooth Fairy, and when we assumed our parents knew everything and could certainly provide a shield of protection against even the fiercest attacks. For those of us who grew up in less than ideal situations, there was hope that simple, easy answers involving magic beans or potions could take care of dilemmas like financial shortages or troubles within our parents' relationships.

Many adults believe that preserving any of the magic and awe we once knew means we are still childish and naive. There is a temptation to cast away all of what made Neverland special, like some jacket we outgrew long ago. But while we realize the Earth is not flat and it is highly unlikely we will encounter fairies in the glen, we should still carry a part of the underlying spirit of some of these stories and beliefs. After all, these tales give life meaning and purpose. They involve notions like the world is basically a good place and that while humanity is flawed in many ways, we sustain the hope that we can and will do better. We need to trust that good ultimately triumphs over evil, both in our own hearts and psyches and in the world at large. For some, these are the strangest Neverland tales of all, but they are ones that we desperately still need to believe, even as adults.

It is so difficult for adults to keep believing after one too many bumps in the grown-up world, and yet this is exactly what we have to do—believe. We have to embrace the whole package of life—the ups, downs, triumphs, and losses—and still carry in our hearts the notion that a special magic worth experiencing is present in all of these. To hold on to these notions gives adults courage to open their hearts to others and allows them to show their children that a special wonder can still be found in the adult world. Failing to do this leaves many of our spirits broken.

There are inherent dangers in this process of growing up, like becoming disillusioned and making the mistake of leaving *all* the magic of childhood and Neverland behind. Losing our way on these matters makes us think that life is little more than a fierce competition for limited resources, or that we need to advance our political, personal, or religious agendas at the expense of others. If these psychological shifts occur, they leave an adult's life colorless, dull, or even worse. Somehow we have to figure out how to reside in the middle of these challenges and difficulties and still have a good life.

In some cases, we make this challenge of affirming our existence amid life's ups and downs even more difficult by adding unnecessary troubles. Adhering to outdated or dysfunctional social and cultural mores that govern the lives of men can contribute to the dilemma. Many of the commandments suggest we still cling to archaic guidelines for boys and men. A chief example is that being a man is a full-time job. A man's sense of masculinity is present in every avenue of his life, accompanied by the state of constant self-evaluation. Men learn to ask themselves, "Did I do that right?"

at each turn. Life is hard enough; now imagine if, in every aspect of life, you had to discern if you were up to snuff as a man. Some may mistake this as only the preoccupation of caveman types, but in reality, many men wrestle with this dilemma, and it takes a toll.

These gender-specific challenges place some men at risk for becoming bitter, jaded, or just plain lost. In this chapter, we'll look at "Lost Boys," men who got off track and have lost connection with their sense of authenticity and purpose entirely. Lost Boys appear lifeless and overburdened in adulthood because they have separated themselves from the magic of living. Often they seem emotionally checked out from their jobs and relationships. The aim of this chapter is to help Lost Boys find their way back so they can live meaningful lives.

## The Neverland Barrier

The Neverland barrier, as we saw in the previous chapter, is the imaginary line that separates the world of a child from that of an adult. We discussed how some men can get stuck in Neverland and fail to realize the adult responsibilities and joys of work and love. The full-blown Peter Pan Man has not yet crossed the Neverland barrier in the significant areas of his life; with other men who are less affected, there are only some areas in which they need to grow up. It is important to compare the Peter Pan Man to the Lost Boy on a couple of different points.

It is the act of crossing the Neverland barrier that allows a Peter Pan Man to grow up, while the Lost Boy crosses it too soon and under harsh circumstances. The Lost Boy is either pushed through the Neverland barrier before he is emotionally ready, or he crashes through it because of circumstances beyond his control. The result of this disorienting experience is that he becomes truly lost—lost to himself and his personal truths. A man's individual truths can be thought of as his internal compass, a guide for every aspect of his life. When the compass points "true north," that is, when a man is able to pay attention and follow his own beliefs (while at the same time not being oblivious to the influence of others), his life feels on course. He lives by the true-north self, his inner world of principles guiding him rather than the whims of society or others.

It is important to note that sometimes life events and challenges can affect a man's internal compass. For instance, sometimes when crossing the Neverland barrier, the compass is thrown off just a few degrees and is easily corrected. In fact, growing up is, by its very nature, disorienting to one's internal guidance system. Some of the awkwardness of adolescence, for example, involves not really knowing what you believe or who you are. Kids at this stage try on different personas in what seems like a nonstop shuffle of personalities; the hope is they will find the one that fits in a real way.

Part of the mission at this stage is to separate from what you have been told by family and society and find out what you really believe. This process is central to becoming your own person, with your own collection of values and beliefs. But there is a built-in disorientation that goes along with reaching this point, and this is a result of distancing yourself from what is known and familiar in order to find your own path. All of this is a normal part of growing up. In fact, going through these types of challenges can help hone and solidify personal truths so that next time, in the face of adversity, the compass is less likely to go off course as much and can be reoriented to its true position more quickly.

Unfortunately, men who eventually become Lost Boys experience a more lasting impact from life events, and this keeps their internal compasses from reorienting to their true directions. They are not the normal adolescent lost-in-the-wilderness phases that almost everyone goes through. Lost Boys have something extra added to their experience that makes things worse. They undergo a series of trials that are beyond their comprehension and are powerfully disorienting on an emotional level; because of such events, these boys can become truly lost to themselves—to what they think, feel, and believe. Unfortunately, in the world of becoming a man, many life occurrences can bring about this state of being.

In his memoir *Where Rivers Change Direction*, Mark Spragg writes about growing up in Wyoming and working for his father on a ranch. His experiences included the joy of being around horses, the beauty of nature, and also learning to be a man. But sometimes he was assigned duties that he was not ready for, and these left a mark. One of the sources of income on the ranch was providing visiting hunters the chance to shoot big game. For game like bears, they used a technique known as "baiting," which involved leaving food to lure the bear to where it could be shot from a safe distance.

On some occasions, a dead horse was left to rot in the designated area. One day, fifteen-year-old Mark was asked by his father to lead a horse to the meadow where it was to be sacrificed. The horse in question was his horse—Socks—the old bay that was his companion and had provided nothing but steady work for many years but was now on his last leg, literally, as a wound to his leg had turned gangrenous. Mark guided his horse to the meadow in what seemed like a funeral procession, chambered a shell in his rifle, and put down his horse as he fought back tears.

When a boy crosses the Neverland barrier in such a rough fashion, his internal compass is thrown out of whack. It no longer points true north; it may just spin and spin, giving inaccurate guidance for the direction of his life. This has an impact on his sense of what he holds as truth and how that guides his steps toward achieving goals and meaning. We need our underlying principles and values; whether we consciously or unconsciously realize it, they direct us in moments of inspiration and desperation. For some, events like these promote a strong desire to purchase a foolproof insurance policy, guaranteeing complete safety.

I remember when I was actively studying martial arts and the occasional new student would show up at the studio. After the prepared lesson for the day, the new student would linger after class with a puzzled look in his eyes. He would ask about the technique that we studied, and then the conversation would slowly turn into a long drawn-out "what if" game. The new student would ask the instructor, "Well, what if someone grabbed you in this way instead, what would you do then?" or, "What if you were in a cramped, dark alley and couldn't do what you suggested? What would you do then?"

or, "What if there were three attackers instead of one? What then?" This line of questioning could seemingly go on forever and reach degrees of absurdity.

Students who seemed particularly anxious often could not let go of this "what if" line of thinking. They wanted an absolutely ironclad guarantee that they would be protected from the world; but, of course, no one could honestly make such an offer. At some point, the instructor would give his pat answer, saying that their likelihood of being able to defend themselves in a difficult situation increased by continuing to train and study. I could see the look that appeared in some of these students' eyes, something akin to, "What do you mean, increase the chances of protecting myself? You are asking me to play the percentages? Isn't there a hotline number I can call in case of emergencies?"

When we discuss the hard realities of the world, and the hope of trying to help children (whether boys or girls), the same pat answer the martial arts instructor gave applies here as well: the likelihood of being able to deal with difficult situations in life increases if you continue to train and study. That is, study your child and the situation, make appropriate interventions, and have suitable discussions. When the harshness of the world creeps into places that are beyond your control, there is one other thing to do: sit with the person who has felt the brunt of the world, hold his hand, and make the commitment: "I will be with you through this." Though you cannot prevent the world from being what it is, at times you can help clean up the mess afterward. Do this in conjunction with trying to take preventive steps to keeps boys from becoming Lost Boys. Remember, Lost Boys are created when harsh events occur that are beyond their reckoning and when there is no one there to help clean up the mess afterward.

## Adult Men as Lost Boys

Lost Boys in adult form may seem like the walking dead. They are physically present but emotionally checked out. This is seen in their relationships with their partners, kids, or even at work. A great example of what a Lost Boy looks like is found in the film *City Slickers*. Billy Crystal plays Mitch Robbins, a man whose moping and complaining alienates everyone in his inner circle. He seems lifeless in his marriage and with his kids, and at work his boss holds a meeting to try to understand what is wrong with him. We see the extent of Mitch's Lost Boy status when he goes to his kids' school for a father's version of show-and-tell to discuss what he does for a living. Much to the horror of both the children and the teacher, Mitch begins to tell how awful and meaningless life is, how existence is downhill after forty, and the best thing you can look forward to is spending your golden years in a nursing home where you mistake one of the attendants for your mother.

At his wife's urging, Mitch and his two best friends go out West to a dude ranch in an attempt to sort out their respective lives. During the ensuing cattle drive, Mitch rethinks some of the things he has carried into adulthood that affect his Lost Boy status. He meets Curly, a frightening relic of a cowboy, who holds up his index finger and declares this is the meaning of life. Curly tells Mitch to find the one thing that matters and everything else will fall into place or to the wayside. The trick is to know what that "one thing" is, because it is different for everyone. From a Lost Boy perspective, that one thing is the internal compass that gives you direction: it is what makes your internal compass point true north again. A Lost Boy has forgotten or lost touch with what this "one thing" is, and without that anchor point, he loses his way.

Sometimes a man drifts slowly into the Lost Boy status, while other times discernible life events are the starting point from which a normal, functioning man goes astray. These triggers can be bitter divorces, career upheaval, or the death of a loved one. In all these cases, a man's meaning and purpose feels ripped away, leaving him short-circuited in his ability to function.

I worked with a client once who was in his fifties and had grown children. He was a bright, honest, and hardworking individual. Unfortunately, he suffered a debilitating injury at a job site and was forced to go on disability. Before his injury, he was working toward becoming an architect and had dreams of providing for his family in a way that his own father was unable to; after his injury, he sank into a deep depression for a number of years before coming to therapy. Due to his disability he was unable to provide for his family in the way he had hoped. In fact, his grown children helped out financially, much to his chagrin. He was challenged to rethink his role as provider. Could he still feel good about being a man even if it meant not being able to provide for his family?

Over the course of therapy, he had much grieving to do. A central part of his problem was feeling that his children would not admire him and, even worse, not respect him because of his financial circumstances. He felt like less of a man because the version of masculinity he grew up with stated explicitly that "provider" was the key role for a man in his family. Because he held this attitude so strongly, his relationships with his children and wife were adversely affected; he felt like a failure, and his resulting depression kept others at bay.

For instance, one Christmas he did not have money to buy presents for his adult children. By his own account, they did not honestly seem too affected by this but gratefully brought him and their mother small gifts. On Christmas day he said he felt so ashamed that he refused to open the presents. He said he would hang on to them and only unwrap them when he could return the favor and buy gifts for them. While the client seemed to feel justified in this rather self-punishing behavior, he also cast a shadow on the holiday experience for his kids, as most of them broke into tears. This was a very telling example of how this man's own conflict about being a man placed a self-imposed barrier between him and his family.

The good news about these types of stories is that men who have become Lost Boys can find their way back. Sometimes this is a long process, but it can be done. It involves rediscovering the meaning and purpose in their lives. This is not an easy thing to do when it has been lost or feels stolen. Large strides can be made by reconnecting to the authentic part of themselves. Sometimes this involves discovering joy and, other times, by cleansing grief.

---

### WAKE-UP CALL:
### *Identify a Lost Boy*

An important point to keep in mind is some Lost Boys already carry a burden from growing up male. There may be a predisposition to lose touch with their authentic selves because their training as males sent them down that path. With each step away from their true path, their needed resources were further depleted. They cannot be the man you want them to be if they are not connected to their source of authenticity. Below are five key descriptions of a Lost Boy:

Lost Boys have crashed through the Neverland barrier, leaving them disoriented.

They have lost the ability to feel things and are often numb inside.

Lost Boys have lost touch with their authentic sense of being—their compass does not point true north.

Lost Boys have lost a sense of purpose and meaning.

Lost Boys often look like the living dead.

---

## Attunement

Psychologists have long noted the importance of "attunement." While this concept has varying definitions and subtle nuances, we refer to it as being in-sync with how another thinks or feels and responding in kind. Being attuned does not necessarily mean you are in full agreement with the other person, but rather that you can understand where they are coming from and handle that knowledge with sensitivity. In the best sense, attunement provides the psychological sense of accompaniment as another explores his or her feelings and thoughts. The potential rewards of attunement include facilitating another's self-exploration and growth as well as deepening the sense of emotional connection between two people.

Attunement has direct implications for a wide variety of settings including being a model for how a caregiver interacts with his or her children. A child's self-awareness and sense of self are enhanced by the right level of attunement. Psychoanalyst Donald Winnicott discussed how a caregiver needs to be aware of a child's earliest expressions of authentic personality. A caregiver's attunement helps the child's "true self" continue to grow. While attunement has been a particular focus for the health and welfare of infants and children, this same concept is important for adults. Attunement is a necessary part of vibrant adult interactions that range from good friends and romantic partners to the healing power of the therapeutic relationship. In terms of the latter, psychoanalyst Heniz Kohut suggested that one aspect of attunement, empathy, was the major tool of psychoanalysis. Empathy refers to the ability to think and feel oneself into someone else's inner world.

Each of us has an ongoing flow of inner experiences made up of thoughts, feelings, hopes, desires, frustrations, disappointments, and so forth. In order to understand the complex inner world of another person, one has to have some firsthand knowledge of the other's moment-to-moment happenings. Empathy accomplishes this task. As one gathers information from enough of these empathic moments, thus perceiving what another person thinks or feels in particular situations, what might have been the cloudy world of another begins to unfold and take shape. One begins to understand what prompts a person to feel or act a certain way. This form of attunement is particularly helpful in adult relationships, especially regarding the complicated issues of work and love.

Most all of us have had the experience of trying to put into words an experience or feeling that is complex and unclear. It could be about a job or relationship, or in one instance, a friend's anxiety when showing up at lunch. He told me that his preteen son was trying out for the local soccer team and had yet to hear the results. My friend couldn't really understand why he was so anxious—after all, his son wasn't. He began reminiscing about how soccer was an important part of his own formative years and even played a pivotal role in courting his wife. It also helped define him as a man and the way he "worked well with others." Even now, he and his son would create new soccer games in the backyard, his son making playful comments about beating him at these when he "got old." "When will that be?" he would ask his son. "Oh, about five years." When my friend missed a shot, his son would adjust that time frame by six months or so. As we talked through lunch, it was becoming clear that soccer was a complex issue for him, not just about a game but a way of connecting with others. He feared that avenue of relating would somehow be taken away if his son did not make the team and decided to pursue some other interest

There are also more advanced attunement skills in which a person not only understands but also takes action by validating or explaining the inner world of another. For example, an attuned individual might say to another: "It makes sense to me that you feel that way, because you see the world [or relationships, or yourself] from this perspective." This approach is used in a number of situations ranging from offering support to those who have had a tough day to helping another really define who they are as a person.

As we will see throughout this book, these forms of attunement provide a sense of safety but also supply the emotional fuel for potential growth and change. Psychologist Daniel Stern stated that certain types of attunement actually involve "changing the other by providing something the other did not have before or, if it was present, by consolidating it." That is, attunement can actually transform a person for the better by increasing their self-understanding or providing them a nurturing or corrective experience. After all, when people are more aware of the perspective from which they operate, or suddenly feel more complete as people, they can make choices to adjust their point of view and its accompanying actions.

Attunement ultimately provides a fundamental psychological need that both genders require for a healthy life. It is an active process that requires concentration and practice. Just like any other type of skill set, there is a wide range of variability regarding how easily someone develops the skills of attunement. However, the effort is worth it. And you thought all you were doing was "just listening"! The next section highlights how these skills of attunement are used in the role of the "repackager."

# The Repackager

Once a friend shared with me the story of his mother's passing. "Was it expected?" I asked. "My father knew she was going to die, but not me. I was only seven at the time." At that age, you don't have the life experience to know that people really die. Or, if you do, you know that somehow you are magically protected from it, as are all the members of your immediate family. (Well, maybe not your little brother, because he is mean.) My friend went on to say, "I wish my father would have taken me somewhere to talk with someone. You know, a counselor or something." "Did he talk about it with you?" I asked. "No," he said, "my father just got busier with work. There were a lot of medical bills to pay, and he wanted to make sure we didn't lose our house. So he spent a lot of time away from the home he was trying to save. He has regretted it for the past twenty years." "What about you?" I asked. "Well, she has been gone for a long time; I guess you learn to live with it."

In this situation and those like it, there does need to be someone who helps sort through the messiness of loss and difficult events. True, you can learn to "live with it," but that is not the same as having peace. The "living with it" solution is based on the idea that time heals all wounds. Sadly, that is not the case. If you don't work through the underlying loss or conflict, the only thing time does help with is your ability to distance yourself from it. After so many months or years, you are left with the impression that it is all squared away; that is, until you find yourself weeping indiscriminately at Kodak and Hallmark commercials.

When life's difficulties cannot be avoided, a "repackager" is needed to offset things. A repackager is someone who can help you look at a situation that is beyond your control or emotional comprehension and make better sense of it. They can offer solutions and strategies when you are dead in the water, not knowing what to do or how to proceed. A repackager also "contains" painful emotions. This means they don't shy away from hearing what is troubling you. This is no small task—holding fast in moments when people reveal the raw pain that has short-circuited their functioning takes maturity. They really hear your story, running it over in their minds until they are in tune with the situation and how it affects you. In a sense, they have the aerial view of what's going on but can also zoom in on all the small details.

A repackager does another thing: because they are outside of the situation and more in touch with their own resources, they help a person literally "repackage" the emotional events that have been so overwhelming. They can then present back to the other person the situation in a way that is more manageable. I do not mean they sugarcoat it or distort what has happened, but instead they help you sort through it. In short, a repackager's function is to help people make peace with their pain.

Imagine that someone comes to you after a rough experience with some normal or out of the ordinary life event. It is as if they show up at your doorstep with a cardboard box that represents the experience they just had. The contents of the box represent the raw feelings, thoughts, and troubles of the incident. If you are a good repackager, your first task is to invite the person to open the box and share what is inside. This involves being willing to hear someone go through each of the items in the box and allowing them to explain and explore what each means to them. When folks do this they sometimes feel very emotional; they may weep or get angry. There is a reason this package does not sit peacefully. There are many troubling things inside. For some, the opportunity to talk about the contents of the package will be enough help, but part of being a good listener and repackager entails going further by asking questions about a particular item in the box: "How did that feel when that happened?" or "How has that affected your life since?"

The next step a repackager takes is to help sort through the items in the box. Some of these contents may need to be reshuffled, packed differently, or taken away entirely if the box is to be closed properly. A good repackager understands and explains how all the items fit—or equally important, don't fit—together. Sometimes a repackager may refer to the many heavy items in the box and convey how they understand the impact they carry. They may also explain how it makes sense that this box couldn't fit in the closet very easily, because it still needs some re-sorting; these two skills of understanding and explaining the contents of the unsorted box can be powerfully helpful and healing.

A repackager's main purpose is to help someone make peace with a difficult life event. As a therapist, that is one of my main functions: help people repackage the events of their lives that cause them trouble. My goal is to help the people I work with find as much peace as they can with the unsorted boxes they have in their lives. Sometimes the box needs to be closed and reopened on a number of occasions and over a given period of time.

As a parent, partner, daughter, or wife, you can be a repackager for the men in your life. This involves dealing with boxes that appear in relation to day-to-day events, like bad days at work or struggles within the family. Other times more extreme situations create packages that may take longer to work through. Sometimes old boxes that have been waiting to be reopened for a long time sit out of view but not in a peaceful spot. Some of these were the original causes of the Lost Boy losing his way. These boxes are marked "Fragile, handle with care." My guess is that you've already been functioning as a repackager and have not even been aware of the help you've been giving.

# Repackaging the Troubles of Boys and Men

As a kid, even in normal circumstances, you need the attention and presence of a repackager. You need someone to make sense of a world you don't understand, someone who can look beyond the overwhelming situation

and help sort through it when you have reached the limits of your emotional knowledge and comprehension. Repackaging may be necessary in all
types of situations, like when the family pet dies, or when you need to
explain why the little child on TV is bald from cancer treatment, or when
Mommy and Daddy decide to divorce. If this repackaging is not done, these
events remain unprocessed, and this may create a Lost Boy.

A repackager is especially needed for little boys who begin to feel the
weight of their man-training. Even in homes that encourage their son to be
his own man from early on and do not teach the traps of the Ten
Commandments of Growing Up Male, repackaging is still necessary.
Sometimes children come home and wonder why they are different from
other boys, or why "so-and-so" at school made fun of them. Tom's son
Derek seemed to show early on that he was a sensitive and creative boy.
What Derek liked to do best was draw and make up stories. He was naturally attuned to others in distress and tried to comfort them. Sometimes,
when his sensitivity overwhelmed him, Derek became the one who needed
to be consoled.

Derek had a younger sister who, by comparison, was a rough-and-
tumble girl who showed no fear. She was much more like her father than
Derek in that way. Tom, though tempted to make comparisons between his
son and daughter, worked hard to sit on those reactions. He wondered,
"Should I toughen Derek up? After all, the world is not a friendly place.
Will he be eaten alive by other kids at school?" But at the same time he was
aware that this was who Derek was, a sensitive, creative young boy. To try to
squelch that part of him would be changing who he really was at the core
of his being. Nevertheless, kids teased Derek for a version of this very thing,
calling him a "baby" for being too sensitive.

Tom decided that he would continue to encourage Derek's sensitivity
and creativity, but also teach him how to handle kids who might tease him.
Sometimes Tom would help take the edge off of Derek's day if something
happened at school. He would reinforce the idea that Derek's creativity and
sensitivity were gifts; they were what made Derek his own unique person.

Tom also told Derek that not everyone had the same gifts and that some others kids might not always understand. Derek could learn a way to not take himself or the other kids so seriously when they didn't understand him. He could use his creativity in the form of humor to playfully laugh at himself at times, and even share that humor with other kids.

Even though it was not easy at first, Derek learned this important skill. Other kids saw that he looked comfortable in his own skin. He seemed secure enough to make good-natured fun of himself. Other kids felt drawn to this creative kid who could deal with his own insecurities. In the end, Tom did not encourage Derek to be someone he was not. Instead, he taught his son how to enhance his natural creativity and sensitivity. As a repackager, Tom did some important things for Derek: (1) He helped make an unbearable situation more tolerable, (2) He offered new perspectives and strategies, and (3) He contained his son's difficult emotions. All of these abilities can be applied in raising boys or helping adult men.

Sometimes, when there is significantly more damage from the past, a repackager has some tough work to do. In the movie *Good Will Hunting,* Will Hunting (played by Matt Damon) is a brilliant but troubled young man who is court-mandated to see a psychologist because of repeated public fighting. The initial part of the relationship with the psychologist (played by Robin Williams) is very bumpy, as Will uses all types of emotional defenses to keep from revealing vulnerable areas.

Through the patient help of the psychologist, Will shares his troubled past, including his history of abuse by his father. Will's father would give him the choice of what he wanted to be beaten with: a belt, chain, or wrench. Will did what most people living in a chronically abusive situation would do: in order to feel safe, he used all manner of ways to keep others at an emotional distance. These coping skills followed him into adulthood. Sometimes he put on a tough, self-reliant pose or pretended to be the underachieving, indifferent rebel. Other times he just wanted to feel invisible; after all, he couldn't be hurt if he couldn't be seen.

At an even deeper level, he tried to make sense of how a parent could do such things to a son. Parents didn't hurt their kids in this way unless they deserved it, right? He believed that if he had been a better kid, or smarter, or better behaved his father wouldn't have abused him. The sad part is that while Will's abuse had nothing to do with his shortcomings or worth, from the emotionally arrested perspective of a Lost Boy, he could not hold to any explanation other than blaming himself.

The pivotal scene in the movie occurs when the psychologist realizes Will still blames himself for the abuse. He tells Will, "It is not your fault." Will puts him off by putting up his defenses, but the psychologist repeats, "Son, it is not your fault." He moves closer into Will's space and says it again, "It is not your fault." Finally, this breaks through and touches a place inside of Will. Someone was actually standing up for him, telling him he deserved better than the abuse he had received. He begins to realize that the abuse was not his fault and starts down the road toward his new identity: "Good Will Hunting." The psychologist in this situation challenged Will, knowing how difficult the confrontation would be for both of them. He supported Will by shielding him from his own self-incriminating thoughts and feelings.

Being a repackager is not easy work. This is especially the case when there are damaging experiences that short-circuited the Lost Boy's emotional functioning and sent his compass spinning. Repackaging is more than just easy, warm, experiences. Sometimes it involves immense strength. We will look at this more closely in Chapter 11 when we discuss what it means to be a "guardian."

# The Cures for Lost Boys

One of the difficulties with self-help books is that they usually present a one-size-fits-all solution. Those who read these books sometimes feel frustrated because this all-encompassing approach is not tailored to the needs of the individual. As we have discussed in this chapter and throughout this book, men are not all carbon copies of each other; they vary in terms of differing life histories, things that have affected them, and the resources and limitations they may have. Keeping these individual differences in mind, I would like to offer three different approaches targeted toward helping Lost Boys get on track. All three of these involve transforming Lost Boys into Renaissance Men.

In many myths and traditions around the world, there is a belief in a "birth-death-rebirth" cycle. For instance, ancient man, who farmed and raised crops, recognized there were definable seasons of growth, death, and rebirth. In ancient Egypt, grain, a staple of the Egyptian diet, was personified as a god who was born, grew to its proper height, and then was harvested. Egyptians saw the mystical wonder of the dying god coming back to life the next growing season.

This birth-death-rebirth cycle can be applied to cultures as well. When the ancient Roman Empire fell in 476 CE, budding Western civilization plunged into the Dark Ages, where cultural gains were not only halted but actually regressed. This period of darkness lasted until the advent of the Renaissance Age in the fourteenth century. This marked the reemergence of Western culture. Renaissance actually means "rebirth." In this case, Western civilization was reborn. This rebirth set the stage for today's modern society.

Sometimes the birth-death-rebirth cycle is also apparent on a personal level, when people rediscover the joy of work in a new job or career, or in relationships, where there is an ebb and flow of varying levels of connection and intimacy. Sometimes, relationships that feel like they have grown cold or listless can experience a rebirth as well.

A Lost Boy turns into a Renaissance Man by following the birth-death-rebirth cycle. A Renaissance Man is a reborn man—a Lost Boy who is in the process of finding his way back to himself. A Renaissance Man is a former Lost Boy who is now a healthier, happier, and content man; he has experienced the bumps of life that once led him astray but is now back on course and enjoys the wisdom obtained from working through his prior emotional wounds and Lost Boy status. Having crashed through the

Neverland barrier of the adult world too soon or under harsh conditions, he must go back and cross this barrier once again, only this time under more favorable circumstances. A man does this by revisiting some of the painful events that turned him into a Lost Boy (notions such as what it means to be a man, putting loss in a proper perspective, and so on).

In the caring environment of a relationship with a loved one, therapist, or friend, a Lost Boy can return to where he first began, before he lost his way. Certain events and people may need to be discussed. Life events and recollections may need to be repackaged. This process can be painful and time-consuming. It may take many trips back and forth across the Neverland barrier to gain a lasting peace, but each trip allows a Lost Boy to carry a bit of himself forward, reclaiming who he is. Below are three important approaches for helping the Lost Boy become a Renaissance Man: (1) rediscovering the Eternal Boy, (2) finding his true-north self, and (3) service to others.

## Rediscovering the Eternal Boy

Over the past two chapters we have seen the delicate balance of a man staying in touch with, while not being overpowered by, his spirit and connection with life. For instance, the Peter Pan Man is tempted to let his spirit run wild and not grow up; his unbridled zest for life transforms him into a man-child. If he does not know how to guide this force, it will cause trouble in the areas of work and love.

On the other hand, as in the case with the Lost Boy, his spirit is broken through harsh circumstances. He feels depleted from the difficulties he has encountered. He appears lifeless. Emotionally speaking, a Lost Boy is not whole; he has lost the essential part of his identity responsible for keeping him in touch with his emotions. He does not have that vital connection with feelings that supply the energy to do the many things that need to be done. This can affect his job as well as his relations with those he loves. You might wonder, "If a Peter Pan Man is helped by learning to bridle his spirit in more adult ways, then how can we help a Lost Boy, someone who needs to bring back the spirit of a little boy?"

In the movie *Big*, Tom Hanks plays a boy whose magic wish to be "big" is granted, and he wakes up a grown man. He falls in love, becomes a toy executive, and dances with his boss on the giant keyboard in an F.A.O. Schwartz toy store. He threatens most of his male colleagues because he speaks his mind with no pretense, his boss thinks he is a breath of fresh air because he comes up with creative ideas, and his love interest remarks he is the most grown-up man she has ever known.

There is a Latin phrase, *puer eternus*, which means "eternal boy." The "Eternal Boy" is the name we will use for the Lost Boy who is reconnected to the vital life energy found in the emotional realm. He is revitalized when he reclaims that part of his being. Areas that have lain dormant or dying feel its healing effects. Rediscovering the Eternal Boy brings the gusto back into a man's life; he is playful and energetic again. He may be frisky like a teenager, feel the awe of living in the moment, or experience the power of his feelings as a source of inspiration. He recaptures emotional parts of himself that were lost along the way. Also, being in touch with the Eternal Boy produces high-definition feelings. They may be experienced as more vivid and colorful. This way of experiencing life stems from having all parts of himself present again. And, just like Tom Hanks's character in *Big*, being in touch with the Eternal Boy builds bridges to others, like his children, romantic partner, or business associates and clients. People around the man are often affected by his vitality. They feel the intensity of his connection with the richness of the emotional realm.

A woman once told me the story of when her boyfriend proposed to her. He wanted to visit the place she grew up and the site where her father was buried, realizing how important that relationship was to her. It was wintertime, and after finding her father's grave and sharing a few moments together, he suggested they collect the giant pinecones that hung from the nearby trees. In a few moments she returned and found him down on one knee with an engagement ring in his hand. He was kneeling in front of her father's grave. He said that since her father had passed away and he could not ask for his daughter's hand in marriage in person, he decided that being in his presence was the next best thing. This may be one of the most touching proposal stories I have ever heard. It was authentic and heartfelt. In this moment, this man was very in touch with his Eternal Boy, that part of himself that could appreciate the wonder and joy of the world. One of the important things to keep in mind is that as your partner becomes more connected to his Eternal Boy, you will also benefit.

▶ **Toolbox Tip: Eternal Boy vs. Peter Pan Man**

Let's sort through this concept of the Eternal Boy a bit more by making comparisons with the Peter Pan Man. Both types of men are in touch with the emotional realm that puts vitality into life. They are engaging and draw others to them with their zest for life. The difference is that the Eternal Boy is on the other side of the Neverland barrier, which means these important tools are used in the hands of a grown-up. This is a powerful combination, because the Eternal Boy is both fun and safe.

## The Eternal Boy: Reclaiming Emotion

I have a great deal of respect for authors like Ernest Hemingway and Nick Hornby, who write in honest, declarative language when discussing emotion. They both talk about the emotional realm, but not as some convoluted ride; instead, their prose is effortless, pure, and straightforward. In many ways, men are taught to express emotion in this way—in simple, declarative sentences. This is the result of the commandments and the compression effect of the secret shoe box. When Lost Boys reconnect with themselves, a powerful, emotional honesty is allowed to emerge, and this can be a very touching experience to observe.

The potential cure for a Lost Boy involves men reclaiming a part of themselves that has been lost along the way—their emotional side. Sometimes this distance from feelings is the result of man-training found in the Ten Commandments of Growing Up Male; other times, Lost Boys lose a chunk of themselves as the result of difficult life circumstances. In both of these situations, raw experiences have not been repackaged, so men separate from their feeling-function as a way to cope with painful recollections and emotions. They think, "If I don't allow myself to feel the pain, then it is not there and won't affect me."

This version of the Lost Boy knows that to feel things again will eventually open him up to the painful event(s) that have not been re-sorted. For a man to rediscover the Eternal Boy within himself, he will need to sort through the experiences that led him off track and created his Lost Boy status. In many circumstances, this will involve grief, but the eventual result is the potential to experience other emotions as well, sometimes in a very deep way. We will discuss grief and grieving more in the chapters on "Making Peace with the Past."

## Finding His True-North Self

Some of the most difficult Lost Boy cases are men who have been off course for most of their lives because they were enabled by parents and partners who never allowed them to guide themselves and define life on their own terms. Instead, Lost Boys' emotional growth was stunted due to authority figures (in most cases a parent) who pushed their own hopes, dreams, beliefs, and biases onto their sons. As a result, boys (and men) got off track because they were not using their own internal compasses to guide their lives; instead, they relied on others' notions of how they should be.

When a Lost Boy develops this way, many of their ensuing major life decisions are based on someone else's demands or requests. For instance, a Lost Boy may pursue an education or career because Mom or Dad chose this path for him. This same pattern arises in matters of the heart when men choose partners based on their parents' requirements. Another, contrasting version of this same scenario involves a Lost Boy rebelling against his overbearing parents, who are too involved in his partner selection, by running off with someone he knows will really upset them.

Common to all these scenarios—whether related to work or love—is the fact that the man is not using his own internal guidance system. In one case, he defers, and in the other, he rebels. Neither approach is in accordance with his own true sense of self, that part of him that provides a guide for living an authentic life. We will see the emotional wreckage associated with these types of relationships in Chapter 9.

How do you help someone who has lived most of his life off course, either through never standing his ground or through rebellion? Initially, it is difficult to know where to start, because many of these issues are stuffed deep inside of a man. Not living life from an authentic core is disorienting and deflating. In many instances, a Lost Boy can only recall moments (versus long periods of time) when he was truly being himself.

If these moments happened in the Lost Boy's childhood, they may have occurred under unusual circumstances, like when out-of-town guests were staying over, when he went away for summer camp, or when he visited with friends or relatives. It could be that his authentic self surfaced in a special environment or through a special person, and these instances and brief encounters gave him a much-needed breath of fresh air where momentarily he was in tune with his true-north self, and it felt marvelous.

He may feel like he is on track for the first time in his life, only to find that when he returns to his familiar setting, all the old expectations are still there. The previous "keepers of the internal compass" (parents or the like) may react like, "My, you're acting odd today; not quite yourself." The truth is, he is acting like himself for the first time in his life, and if not recognized as such, that part of him could be squelched.

Relationships with ourselves and others are governed by homeostasis. That is, when a pattern is set, for good or bad, it attempts to maintain equilibrium. This is true for Lost Boys as well. A parent who has trouble keeping his/her own biases in check may react unfavorably to a boy being his own person. The parent may mistakenly label his behavior as deviant, abnormal, rebellious, or uncouth. Extra sanctions are put in place to ensure that the boy does not make the same "mistakes" again. The parent does not realize the harm that is being done by not encouraging him to follow his authentic self. So we see that some Lost Boys misplace their internal compasses early on by not following their true course, while others misplace them later due to certain life events, such as illness, death, divorce, or financial upheaval.

Another version of the Lost Boy can be seen in the midlife crisis. Things may have been building up for a while, maybe over the course of many years, and as they finally reach a boiling point, things come undone. The final trigger that sends him spiraling out of control may manifest itself in job loss, an affair, or the sudden need to take up stock car racing.

While these are all differing scenarios, what is similar is how to get the Lost Boy back on course—he must find his true-north self. For some, this search will build upon the moments from childhood when he was in touch with his authentic nature. He uses these faint memories as a guide, but the real task is to find the environment, atmosphere, and/or connection with himself or others that helps cultivate that same spirit now.

I believe people have an innate ability to orient themselves to who they really are, just like a compass naturally points north. The difficult part is not getting the compass to point in the right direction but rather clearing away all the junk that prevents the needle from moving back to where it is already inclined to go. For some men, as they sort through the painful legacy of the past, they find that the needle moves slowly back into the right place.

Mark, a friend of mine at the university, had left teaching several years earlier and taken a full-time administrative role. While there were some benefits, such as a higher salary, for the most part he felt listless and unhappy in his new job, and he was not entirely sure why. Mark's reactions were clearly tied to his present situation, but they hinted at things from the past; some of the issues at work were reminiscent of childhood dynamics, like not feeling that he could speak his mind without repercussions, and subsequently withdrawing and feeling blue. Once he realized this pattern and corrected it at work, he was able to take control of his life and tune in to his authentic self. He thought about going back to full-time teaching and experimented with this notion by volunteering to teach a class. I happened to walk by his class one day by accident and quietly observed for a few moments. The man was truly in his element.

Mark is Celtic, and I remarked to him later what an "Irish lather" he seemed to be in as he taught—that look in his eyes, his gestures, the sheer intensity of being fully engaged while teaching. He knew he was on the right track by going back to the classroom because of the marked contrast with that of being a full-time administrator. He had rediscovered his true-north self, which in turn led to other positive changes in his life. Because he did not have to continually burn up psychic and emotional energy trying to force himself into a job that didn't fit, he felt freed up to pursue the things he once enjoyed.

## ▶ Toolbox Tip: True-North Self

The true-north self has to do with a man living in accord with his authentic sense of identity. The Lost Boy who has been off course must learn how to reorient his compass to point in the direction that is in keeping with who he really is. Once he has discovered areas of his life that feel on track, he can compare those with ones that have not, or do not, now work. This comparison creates a tangible way of knowing when he is following his true-north self. He may discover that when he is in keeping with the direction of his own compass, his work seems to be more rewarding. Likewise, in relationships with partners, kids, and friends, being himself allows for more meaningful and fun interactions.

## ▶ Toolbox Tip: Adult Summer Camp

You may have noticed that a growing part of the travel and leisure industry caters to adults who are trying to live out their childhood fantasies. This can involve things like going to rock and roll camp, spring training with sports stars from a favorite team, or various types of adventure travel.

Picking the right type of fantasy camp can help the Lost Boy find his way back home. He may tap into long-forgotten fantasies that really energized him as a boy. Choosing to interface with this part of himself again can get him in touch with his true-north self.

## Service to Others

Finally, the third part of transforming from a Lost Boy into a Renaissance Man involves service to others, or working for the greater good. A Lost Boy revisits some of his own past struggles while helping others who are currently wrestling with theirs. There is truth to the notion that teaching, parenting, guiding, or mentoring others can be a rich form of healing and personal growth. A Lost Boy on his way to becoming a Renaissance Man may lend a hand to someone who is preparing for their initial crossing (or recrossing, as when helping a fellow Lost Boy who is a grown man) through the Neverland barrier.

A Renaissance Man can help copilot someone else's journey through the Neverland barrier. They can draw from their own experiences about what worked—and what did not—when helping someone else make it through this potentially treacherous zone. On the outside, it may appear as though the apprentice is the only one gaining from this interaction, since conversations may be more one-sided and focused on the other person's issues and concerns. I think this is part of the reason some men are initially turned off by the notion of being a mentor or even becoming a parent—what lingers in their minds is, "Hey, what's in this for me?"

But in truth, when you have experienced your own bumps in the road, there is a deep satisfaction in helping someone else cross the Neverland barrier in a safer, more successful way. It is as if you are experiencing the *birth* of another when they cross the Neverland barrier. In these moments, the Lost Boy on his way to becoming a Renaissance Man begins to think beyond himself, or at least beyond the woes he has experienced. There is a purpose or meaning greater than himself that he begins to serve. He stops looking at the gain/loss column of the balance sheet and instead re-surrenders himself, along with his ego, to the higher purpose that he embraces. If a man fully accepts this mission of helping another, it can be transforming. It can literally change a Lost Boy into a Renaissance Man; he can effect his own rebirth.

Another form of this can occur when a Lost Boy serves a greater purpose or cause that touches others but does not necessarily have a singular face. One of my favorite movies that illustrates this idea is *Lilies of the Field*. Sidney Poitier plays Homer Smith, a wandering and somewhat lost handyman who lives out of his car. He is hired by a group of displaced German nuns who are trying to build a chapel in the Arizona desert. The nuns do not speak much English, and their financial holdings are meager at best. Initially, after each task, the handyman brings his itemized list to the head nun, expecting payment. However, at each turn she instead redirects him to another task aimed at building the chapel. It is easy to see that Homer struggles with the gain/loss column; if he is not being paid, how will he profit by doing this job?

At some point he slowly begins to settle into the mission of working without being paid—at least not in the way he expected. He even takes another part-time job so he can work on building the chapel and still have an income, much of which he spends on groceries for the nuns. As there is no money for labor expenses, there certainly isn't any for building materials either, and it seems unlikely that the chapel will ever be completed. But the community pulls together and folks begin donating what they have, whether lumber, light fixtures from their home, or merely their willingness to help build. Homer embraces his role as the chief architect and builder of the chapel without payment in financial terms. His compensation is of another type, one that transforms him from a Lost Boy into a Renaissance Man.

As a parent or partner who is encouraging your Lost Boy to participate in someone else's life, you may hear your man say, "Well, how am I supposed to help someone else when I can't seem to help myself? Isn't that like the blind leading the blind?" Through service to another, or trying to provide nurturing to someone when you did not receive it yourself, funny things begin to happen in your heart and spirit. It makes you confront your own hopes and wishes that went unfulfilled and the letdowns that followed. Essentially, you begin to face what caused your own Lost Boy status. This becomes an invitation to healing and growth. You fix in your mind that you want to stretch and grow not only for yourself but for those placed in your charge.

Another question a Lost Boy may ask you is "Well, does being a Renaissance Man mean I have to give up my job, shave my head, and give away all my earthly possessions?" Again, you as a partner or parent can convey that service to another in your home or community does not mean that you have to join the Peace Corps, raise kids, or be a mentor. The important thing is to carve out an area where you can give pro bono. Most people know that "pro bono" means you do something for free (it actually means "for the public good"). You do something for the greater good of your community, or those you love, or, even a bigger challenge, those you don't love or may not even know.

### ▶ Toolbox Tip: Creating His EAP

A Lost Boy on his way to becoming a Renaissance Man will need to work on these important tasks, summarized as EAP:

E = Emotional function
A = Authenticity
P = Purpose

Each man must decide, based on his own individual needs, the extent to which he needs to work on these three areas. That is, some men may benefit from time spent on all three, whereas others may target one particular focus.

## ▶ Toolbox Tip: The Map

The following map provides another way to understand the necessary journey of both the Peter Pan Man and the Lost Boy. The Peter Pan Man's task is to cross the Neverland barrier and enter into the adult world of work and love. He starts at point A, which is in the realm of boyhood, and then, through the needed work, matures and enters the grown-up world represented as point B. In contrast, the Lost Boy resides in the grown-up world, point A, but needs to cross back over the Neverland barrier to find a part of himself that has been lost, represented as Point B. This task could involve finding his feeling function, sense of authenticity, or purpose in life. At point C, the Lost Boy then reenters the grown-up world as a Renaissance Man.

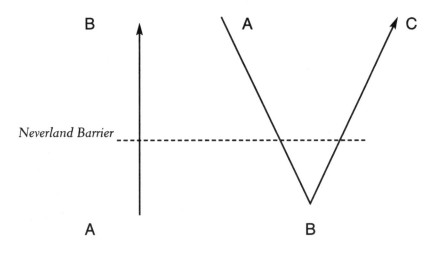

The Peter Pan Man                    The Lost Boy

# Conclusion

Lost Boys are men who have lost touch with their authentic selves. In this chapter we explored three different ways to get back on course, all of which lead to a Lost Boy's new status as a Renaissance Man. The first approach involved reacquainting himself with his Eternal Boy, the wellspring of a man's emotional world that adds richness and color to his life.

In the second approach, we learned how the Lost Boy needs to discover or rediscover his true-north self, which entails recalibrating his internal compass so that it points to his authentic self. When a man follows the lead of his internal compass, it does not ensure that life will be free of challenges and hard times—but he will be better able to weather them because he is doing what feels on course for him. He will be in touch with his emotions to such a degree that when he is off course, he will be able to apply what he has learned to get back on the path in all areas of his life, including his relationships at home and at work.

Finally, the last approach in transforming from a Lost Boy to a Renaissance Man is through service to others, whether as a parent, caregiver, mentor, or volunteer. Transformation occurs when a Lost Boy interfaces with his own painful legacy; he is asked to give to others in ways that he never received himself. This process invites him to heal his own wounds as he attends to those of others. There are many transformative lessons that can be learned on the journey from Lost Boy to Renaissance Man.

# CHAPTER CUES

1. The task of growing up can be challenging; some are tempted to become jaded, bitter, or lost.

2. Lost Boys are men who have lost their connection with their feeling function, sense of authenticity, and/or purpose in life.

3. A Lost Boy's challenge is to become a Renaissance Man and recapture that part of himself that has been lost. He can do so by:

   • rediscovering the Eternal Boy.

   • finding his true-north self.

   • serving others (by assisting other Lost Boys in crossing the Neverland barrier or through service to a higher purpose beyond themselves).

# PART III

# MAKING PEACE
# WITH
# THE PAST

# 7

# The Father and Mother Wounds

In this chapter, we will explore the emotional legacy created from damaging parental relationships. For many men, the troubles attached to these important connections from the past not only impact how comfortably they live in their own skin, they can also unwittingly create adverse interactions in the arenas of work and love. Significant others, children, and business associates can all feel the sting of residual parental wounds left unhealed. Affected behaviors can range from mildly irritating to downright destructive.

"Shadow parents" can be the core cause for many of the troubles that affect people. A shadow parent is an exaggerated or skewed notion of an actual caregiver that a child creates in his formative years. Because shadow parents are formed from a child's perspective, without the benefit of maturity and experience, they are often distorted images of moms and dads. This doesn't mean that the child's notion of his shadow parents is totally untruthful, only that his limited experience in the world does not give him the depth of insight into his parents that he will gain as he becomes an adult. Sometimes the basis of these images are the childlike perceptions and fantasies that we have already discussed in this book, like people should be perfect or belong exclusively to us. Other times, the painful legacy of feeling let down or misunderstood by caregivers complicates and further distorts these images.

Shadow images can form in normal and difficult childhood circumstances, but their degree of distortion and ability to cause disruption in one's life does say something about the psychological conditions in which one grew up. In a normal state of affairs, where emotional needs are met but the usual disappointments are present, images still need to be fine-tuned, progressively mirroring the real people from which they were constructed. Likewise, the accompanying emotional reactions are revised, becoming in tune with a more adultlike perspective. Even with normal situations, sometimes both images and reactions can be intense. As mentioned previously, growing up is difficult enough even in the best situations, affecting how one perceives oneself and others. Some, like psychoanalyst Melanie Klein, believed that obtaining a more realistic perspective of one's internal parental images was work that occupied the entire life span. One of the take-home messages is that making peace with the inner world of shadow images is a task with wide application; for those with even more difficult personal legacies, these images are particularly important to address.

For instance, a child who lives in an unsafe environment, who isn't nurtured, and who may be outright neglected has even fewer tools to take his own parents' shortcomings and history into consideration; he only knows that he is hurt, angry, hungry, and so on, and must find a way to live within his family. Often the difficult legacy of such personal histories is to become much more out-of-focus in terms of perceiving oneself and others, and simultaneously parental images increase in their power to evoke emotional, intense reactions and influence one's behavior.

When I refer to shadow parents throughout this chapter (and others), I am referring to these mental images children have formed in their early years. I use the phrase "shadow parent" because it reminds me of how the ancient Greeks thought of the afterlife. In their mythology, when people died, they went to the underworld where they existed only as shadows of the people they once were. Ancient Greeks referred to the dead as *shades* because they appeared as the silhouettes of people; they were transparent, not fully formed. Shadow parents are not fully formed either, since they have been created from a child's perception during his impressionable, formative years.

We will see that, left unaltered, shadow parents linger in the heart and mind well into adulthood, sometimes with all the intensity with which they were originally created. In the worst case, they can cause devastating effects in a man's life; at the very least, they subtract from the quality of his life. These shadow parent images can keep an adult male from operating with full clarity; decisions are made impulsively to avoid the pain of the past. It is like taking one intense scene out of a movie and playing it repeatedly, achieving the same emotionally heightening and sometimes paralyzing effects.

When shadow parents are still in control, it blocks adults (both men and women) from finding peace with the real caregivers the shadow images are based on. When trying to come to an in-depth understanding of a real parent's limitations in terms of the caregiver/child relationship, it is often crucial to gain a fuller perspective, or the shadowy image of that parent remains the person's sole preoccupation. These frozen images of the shadow parents need to be integrated into a fuller, more honest picture of the true parent if peace is to be found. This tough work involves coming to know Mom and Dad as people in their own right, which includes knowing more of the underlying causes of disappointments and limitations. Only then can the painful past be properly sorted out in the light of compassion and understanding. If the proper work is not done, shadow parents linger as emotionally laden images created from difficult experiences while growing up.

These experiences, which occurred when caregivers left emotional marks due to misunderstandings, shame-filled moments, or various forms of abandonment, often become a lasting part of the psychological and emotional makeup of men (and women). Although the proverb says "Time heals all wounds," we know that the influence of painful scenes from our past do not just dissipate with age. For instance, a patient well into his seventies once told me that going through therapy was the first time in his life he felt some freedom from the shadow image of his father. Until then, he would often picture in his mind's eye the paternal shadow image making critical accusations whenever he made a mistake. This often led him to second-guessing his choices, or worse, made him feel paralyzed in both work and love.

These shadow images are important not just because they stay in our memories such a long time, but also because we carry them with us wherever we go, like a miniature DVD player that always plays the same old family drama. While one is not always aware of the onscreen antics of the shadow parents, they often follow us into many scenarios. They wait in the shadowy recesses of the heart and mind, and in moments of desperation, uncertainty, or disappointment, they spring to life, replaying scenes in what seems like a never-ending loop.

Sometimes this involves reliving a painful recollection, while other times shadow parent images can actually guide a person's behavior or way of relating to others as damaging moments from the past parallel ones in present-day situations. This may occur with one's actual parents, when the same old arguments and conflicts from the past get played out again in the present.

Activating shadow parent images may also include attracting others who resemble shadow parents to revive the role of the original cast member in the well-worn drama. These shadow parent stand-ins can be friends, romantic partners, bosses—anyone who can fill the part.

People can also unwittingly bait others into acting like a shadow parent. For instance, if you have unresolved authority issues related to a parent, chances are those old tapes will begin playing again when similar themes arise, like when someone tries to "boss you around." The connection may not be made that, "Hey, this is exactly how I used to relate to my mom or dad"; however, the same emotional reaction will still surface, setting up old self-destructive patterns. One thing that makes this self-defeating cycle possible is that these scenes have been reenacted so many times that the lines and stage cues are known by heart. Act 1, scene 1: The shadow parent (or a stand-in) enters and says, "Be a man." The boy or man takes his cue and responds as he did when he was a child—with vulnerability and unhealed hurt, anger, or abandonment.

Understandably, shadow parent images elicit strong primal emotions that can be overwhelming. Even grown-ups can feel as though they have turned back the hands of time and reentered their childhood. When this occurs, adults feel stripped of the mature skills and talents they've learned through the years and stand powerless in the presence of the intimidating shadow parent. Since the images of the shadow parent are constructed from the perspective of a child, this often leads to a skewed image, since they do not have a complete picture of the parents' limitations and shortcomings. Children often interpret these parental shortcomings as proof they are unworthy of their parents' love and care, when in reality, many parents are not able to give children what they need because they don't have it themselves.

Directly interfacing with shadow images, even as an adult, causes one to question the legitimacy of one's worth. Nothing undercuts confidence or a sense of personal power like these shadowy images that reside within. This type of pain causes people to duck and cover as quickly as possible, often through destructive thoughts and behaviors. People use their repertoire of survival skills to escape the power of the parental shadow images—drugs, alcohol, impulsive sex, or aggression—something that will make the pain go away quickly, or at least distract them from it.

There is another troubling aspect regarding the shadow parent image: often it not only affects a person's own happiness, but it can have serious effects on others as well. A shadow parent image can cause you to pass on the cycle of disappointing relationships to your children, or it can make life difficult for a significant other, family, and friends. This is why it is imperative to understand more about the shadow parent images and to make peace with them. This will be our mission over the next two chapters.

# The Importance of the Father/Son Relationship

When the Industrial Revolution occurred in the nineteenth century, a once-agrarian society took to the cities to work in the mills and factories. This had a significant impact on middle- and working-class family units. Whereas before all members of the family occupied the same physical space on farmland, now the man spent many hours working away from home. Subsequently, the family unit was divided into two separate spheres based on gender, one for those who toiled in the public world of "work" and one for those who stayed at home. Dad took care of the work world, and Mom took care of hearth and home.

For more than 100 years now, our society has tried to free itself from the influence of this model of a divided sphere of responsibility based on gender. The important thing to draw from this little history lesson is that the division of spheres into work and home duties gave a false impression about what both men and women could accomplish. What did a man know about raising children in a nurturing way? That was the domain of women; they were biologically wired to do that sort of thing, right? And likewise, what did women know about excelling in the world of work? Weren't men following their genetic predispositions by being the breadwinners? Much of this outdated way of narrowly defining all men and women's rights and responsibilities has been challenged and dismissed. The rigid line that was once thought impossible to cross for either gender is much more permeable today. Men can be good nurturers, and women can be first-rate corporate executives.

However, the legacy of the division of spheres still remains in one important area—its impact on raising boys. We still have trouble with the idea that certain characteristics belong exclusively to the domain of one gender. We still hold to the stereotypical laundry list of what it means to be a man: physical toughness, suffering quietly when need be, not letting emotions get the best of us, and so on. When raising boys, who better to teach them how to be a man than other men? In fact, as we have noted in the commandments, a common misconception is that what women "naturally" bring to the table corrupts a boy's sense of masculinity. Boys and men learn to fear all things labeled as feminine.

As the artificial division of spheres based on gender in parenting is slowly removed, we will realize that raising boys is not either gender's exclusive job. But for many men raised in the old school of thought, the legacy of absent fathers or those who did not express love enough still haunts them. This is important, because a boy is taught from early on that someday an older man will teach *him* how to be a man. Without this training, many men feel inadequate or shortchanged in the area of manliness. They may secretly hope that a manual explaining all the things they need to know about being a man will someday come along. This hope has been the basis of many fad masculinities, from the 1970s' sensitive man, to the Marlboro man cowboy, to the more metrosexual man of today. When men feel like they are a couple of steps behind other men, this can weigh on them and subsequently lead them to search for real answers.

Once I gave a talk at a retirement home to male residents whose average age was well into the mideighties. My hope was that the talk on masculinity would encourage them to fill out some questionnaires for a project I was working on. After the talk, a tall, elderly man approached and asked rather sheepishly if he could speak with me privately. This man looked like the prototypical Texan, right down to his cowboy boots and leather vest. He told me in nearly a whisper that he would like to fill out the questionnaire, but there was a problem. He went on to say that he grew up without a father and was afraid that he would ruin my research project if he filled out the survey. What this elderly gentleman was saying to me in so many words was that he felt like his worth as a man was suspect because he did not have a male to guide and validate his being a man. I will never forget the pained look in his eyes. I stood dumbstruck as I watched him walk away. In retrospect, I wish I could have done something to alleviate the burden of pain he had felt for so many years.

Fathers differ in terms of level of involvement with their sons. Some could pick their son out of a lineup but little else. Others occupy the same physical space for years but find themselves lost for words in trying to have conversations beyond that of sports or the weather. Still others learn how to reach across the divide and authentically connect, while some father/son relationships are mired in lifelong conflict. One of the most important relationships you can know about regarding the man you love is the one he shares with his father. A man's relationship with his father is a special thing. It is an aspect of his life that must be put into perspective so he can be truly happy.

A man wants two things from his father. The first is that he will teach him how to be a man. Some "fatherless" men complain that their sense of masculinity is on rocky ground because no one was there to teach them all the nuances of manhood. This includes all the nuts and bolts of what a man does and, equally important, what he does not do. One of my clients who was exploring his notion of how to be a man once stopped midsession in frustration and said, "Look, can we just cut to the chase and you just tell me how I am supposed to be as a man?"

The second thing a man wants from his father is his blessing. This is a high psychological priority for men, feeling that their father can look at them and say, "Son, you are a good man and I am proud of you." You may be surprised by the number of successful, accomplished men who still carry around the wound of not having a father's blessing. It haunts them. They wonder how so many other people in the world can see their worth and value yet their father seems unable to. They hold out on giving themselves the self-approving nod because Big Daddy didn't. In the following section, we'll look at ways to put these two wishes to rest.

## Becoming a Man

When I was at a conference a number of years ago, I ran into an old colleague who was brimming with excitement. He was a member of a "weekend warrior" men's group. He was in his fifties, well educated, and very bright. He said that he had recently become an "elder" in his men's group and now had the ability to bless younger men and help them become men. Younger than him by a number of years, I was not sure if he was implying he would like to "bless me," if he thought my sense of masculinity needed to be initiated, or he was just happy about his new status. In any case, I asked him what they did in these elaborate ceremonies out in the woods. He replied that it was very secret and that I would have to come to one of the gatherings to experience it firsthand.

Looking back on that encounter, I remember feeling a bit puzzled and thinking the whole thing was a little strange. While I am a firm believer in the power of rituals and their potential to help with transformation, they have to be personally meaningful to the individual. I knew that standing out in the woods with a procession of male strangers "blessing me" would not really help me with my sense of masculinity; yet, the underlying spirit of this ceremony seemed focused on healing the hurts that many men had experienced due to the lack of a father's approval or teaching on how to be a man. Without someone to say, "You have arrived as a man," it is hard to know when you have achieved that status.

Searching for the definable event or period in men's lives that officially marked the entrance into manhood sounds appealing. It acts as a tangible and alluring starting point because we want to believe that by simply enacting certain rites and rituals, we will suddenly gain a solid sense of our masculinity. But in reality, these types of initiation ceremonies do not really create the psychological sense of being a man; rather, they act as a point of crystallization for men. That is, all the events that shape one's masculinity up to that point reach a sort of critical mass during "rituals." Or, as my colleague would surely agree, these weekend retreats are a beginning point from which to build. Maybe the potential healing in these ceremonies and those like it comes from the willingess of men to gather with others to search for identity and experience a shared sense of community.

Some men may recall those essential moments when they felt like they became a man. This may be when they stood up to an overbearing parent for the first time, made love, or even endured some type of physical trial or tribulation. For them, whatever the defining event—ceremony, ritual, or some specific encounter or triumph—it was the culmination of all the smaller events from the past that led up to that point. Men's sense of masculinity is built step-by-step from infancy onward.

This is important, because a boy does not just become a man overnight. In fact, the pressure to place boys in situations that will make them men (before they are ready) can backfire. Part of becoming a man is about assuming adult responsibilities in the areas of work and love, but some boys are in dysfunctional circumstances and need to assume those responsibilities prematurely.

For instance, a boy with an alcoholic father and a codependent mother might be the one who makes sure his dad doesn't drive drunk, pays the bills, and takes his younger siblings to school. Some boys with absent or abusive fathers find themselves in the position of being the emotional equivalent of surrogate spouses for their mothers. In these instances, young boys are thrust into manhood without really gaining the maturity they need to navigate a grown-up world. As we saw in earlier chapters in the book, this lack of parenting or not learning healthy boundaries and responsibilities in the proper manner when growing up can create Peter Pan Men and Lost Boys.

Ideally, helping a boy become a man should happen gradually, as they become ready to assume more and more adult responsibilities. They shouldn't be given more responsibilities than they can handle. They need people in their lives who can guide them, which leads us to our next topic: role models.

## What Will a Boy Do Without a Male Role Model?

Many single moms raising boys feel a sense of urgency about having some type of male role model involved in their boys' lives. Some married mothers sense that their husbands do not spend enough time with their sons. Such women have also been persuaded into accepting the lingering but outdated blueprint for man-making that still exists in our society, which is essentially this: a boy has to have a male influence in his life or he is in big trouble. This perceived need is so paramount to the male psyche that it is one of the Ten Commandments for Growing Up Male.

The male role model can be a father, uncle, coach, teacher, or big brother. The defining rule is that someone with a penis must be around, or how else will the boy learn to be a man? The importance of the male role model is a pervasive subject in TV and the media. For instance, in the male psychology course that I teach, I show a videotape of *The Simpsons*, the animated family that includes Homer, Bart, Marge, Lisa, and Maggie. In one of my favorite episodes, Homer sets out to make his son, Bart, a man. He sets him in front of a billboard advertising cigarettes with beautiful women engaged in a pillow fight. He takes him to a steel mill to see how real "Joes" work. Finally, he takes Bart hunting, because as Homer's trusted friend remarks, "Nothing will make you a man faster than killing something beautiful." Of course, this is satire at its best, as at each turn Homer's attempts to make Bart "a man" fail.

But is the male role model really the answer for boys in their struggle to become men? Ultimately, I think that the male role model perspective is flawed, for a couple of reasons. First, the male role model's job is really about teaching a boy to imitate someone else's notion of what it means to be a man. Male role models say, "Look, be like this guy or like me and you will be okay." There is no investment in saying to the boy, "I will help you become your own man, a source of strength for the rest of your life." Traditionally, male role models don't help a boy become his own man; instead they give him what is considered a tried-and-true version of manliness that most people will agree on. They may say, "Yes, that is what a man looks like." What happens if that picture of a man doesn't really fit for the boy? The boy is asked to assume a false persona. This guise, his pretending to be someone he is not, will ultimately act as a barrier to more genuine relationships with others.

Another problem with the male role model approach: just because a person has male genitalia does not guarantee he knows what it means to be a healthy man. A boy can be taught some very destructive lessons from a man who hates women or only uses fear or intimidation to deal with others. A very clear example of this occurs in the New Zealand movie, *Once Were Warriors*. The central character in this movie is a father of three children, including a son. The father is street-tough and emulates many of the stereo-typical notions of being a man, yet we quickly see that he misses the mark on many key aspects of healthy masculinity. He is a hard drinker, bullies his children, and beats his wife when she disagrees—all while claiming his status as a man. Ultimately, it is his inability to step away from this twisted perspective of masculinity that eventually causes him to lose his family. If a boy used him as a role model, he'd inherit a legacy of self-loathing, irresponsibility, and violence—hardly a shining example of manhood.

The last issue I have with the male role model perspective is, traditionally speaking, it pressures boys to make significant strides toward a grown-up version of being a man in the formative years. When boys are asked to undertake tasks for which they are not adequately prepared, the results often include lasting conflicts about being a man as well as an accompanying emotional residual. These conflicts begin to show up early in adolescence and are manifest in how boys view the quality of their parental relationships as well. This may surprise some at first, but we need to consider how the commandments influence childrearing practices regarding how both mom and dad relate to their son.

Research that I have conducted, along with other colleagues, in this area asked college men about their relationships with each parent. More specifically, we inquired about the quality of attachment (or way of connecting and relating) to each parent growing up, as well their ability to separate from parents in healthy ways in order to form their own unique sense of identity. In these studies, males' sense of conflicted masculinity (i.e., male gender role conflict) was related to poor (sometimes angry and distrustful) attachments to each parent and difficulty accomplishing a healthy sense of separation; this affected their sense of self and ability to be with others.

What these findings suggested was that college men felt the lasting brunt of going from boys to men too quickly. This man issue had an impact on their ability to develop into their own unique people and shaped their connection and ability to trust each parent.

Likewise, in other research, boys (ages 13–18) showed a concern for achieving many of the quintessential themes related to traditional masculinity and, much to everyone's dismay, also exhibited many of the same resulting conflicts. Boy's with traditional male role-conflicts focused on not showing others too much of their emotional side, especially regarding their private self and when they were hurting. They also felt in danger of being labeled somewhat suspect for behaving too friendly with other males, or even feeling psychological strain about balancing various school, family, and work responsibilities. All of these stereotypical adult male struggles were related to boys' problems with conduct, emotions, and behavior. These findings suggested some boys might be trying on pants that are too big for them, and their version of grown-up masculinity could lead to emotional consequences.

Sometimes, males encounter challenges that are beyond what they are able to handle, regardless of their age. Becoming a man is a lifetime process, with many stages along the way. A man needs to evolve and mature in sync with the new challenges he encounters, and often as an adult, he needs help from others (men and women) who can mentor him.

In place of a male role model, I would suggest a new role: that of a *guardian*. Being a guardian is more than showing a boy a paint-by-numbers way to achieve manhood. Instead, a guardian can be a man or woman whose central role is to be invested in the boy becoming *his own man*. This is a much more labor-intensive commitment than just pointing to a set of man behaviors and telling them to follow that as an example.

A guardian honors the person a boy is becoming without shoving a list of his or her notions of masculinity down the boy's throat. Boys benefit when they have guardians (male or female) who can offer aspects of humanity that the boys can assimilate into their own personalities. They may be inspired by the guardian's behavior or way of doing things, but they know they are not expected to be carbon copies of their mentor in the different areas of life. The spirit of being a guardian is more about having a type of relationship that allows a boy to become his own person. Mothers, wives, friends, and family, regardless of gender, can be guardians for the important males in their lives. (We will look at this more closely in Chapter 10.)

# The Legacy of the Father Wound

I started practicing martial arts when I was in graduate school, studying for about ten years and earning a black belt in a Japanese art called aikido. While derived from lethal martial arts techniques, aikido instead emphasizes neutralizing others' negative aggression in an efficient and non-aggressive way. It is sometimes referred to as a "loving martial art" with an emphasis on redirecting others' energy and attacks in gentle ways. The ultimate aim is to incorporate more of the underlying principles and philosophy into one's life outside the dojo. But as with any skill set, it is not easily done.

One of my teachers was an older man who was an interesting combination of street-smart toughness and a likable warm side. As I trained with him over the years, I saw many who got the martial arts fever, working out in a frenzied way, sometimes bordering on obsession. Students would try to go to several classes a week, read the philosophy of the martial arts, meditate regularly, and even do extra work beyond that. Sometimes this would happen because a person just fell in love with the art, wanting to immerse themselves in it as much as possible, but other times, this had a lot to do with trying to connect with the chief instructor, who was seen as a father figure.

I remember a fellow student who became passionate about his training and tried very hard to connect with the instructor. The student began to rise through the ranks based on his skill as well as his devotion. However, this situation reached a turning point one day when the instructor and he had an intense disagreement. In all honesty, both parties shouldered some of the blame. Rather abruptly, the student dropped out of class, and angry words between them added fuel to the fire. I remember telling my fellow student that disagreements happen and it really wasn't that big of a deal; he should go make peace.

Looking back now, at the time I failed to realize that it really *was* a big deal. I knew that my fellow student had a very turbulent relationship with his own father, and later I realized that my friend was developing more than his martial arts skills during those training sessions. He was trying to make peace with his own shadow father through replaying some of the issues of conflict from the past with his now stand-in parental figure. Before their rift, the connection with the instructor nurtured him. He was on his way to feeling blessed by his new father figure, something that his biological one was unable to do.

The deeper psychological power of receiving someone's blessing is based on the notion that the one offering the blessing is a greater—and sometimes even supposedly perfect—being. This is a different perspective than respecting a person and valuing their acknowledgment. Conceiving of people as perfect places them on a pedestal that heightens their importance and gives them the power to greatly affect the individual. Having some Joe-ordinary-guy offer his praise does not carry the same punch as a perceived greater other. Likewise, to experience the rapture of feeling valued by a perfect person and then have it stripped away is a painful occurrence. When my fellow student had his disagreement with the martial arts instructor, the notion of being separated from this powerful symbolic blessing placed him in the old, familiar place of feeling uncared for.

When I think of that situation now, my wish is that my friend could have come back to class to train in another way, transitioning his father figure from that of a perceived perfect man who met all of his emotional needs to that of a good person with his own human frailty. But to do this he would have to learn not to take his own father's limitations (or those of the father figure) so personally. A father or father figure's inability to give you everything you want, including a carte blanche blessing for being a man, may not be possible.

Often this unrealistic desire stems from a legacy of deep hurt. The search for the perfect father is a futile one. At some point, we must realize that everyone, even fathers (and mothers too), have their limits. Sadly, those whom we want the most from don't always have it to give. This is simultaneously one of the most painful and rewarding realizations that can be made: painful because a man has to give up yet another fantasy of how he would like the world to be and rewarding because he has the chance to learn many things, including compassion for those who are less than perfect—even himself. If men don't make this transition, they will likely replay this same disappointing scenario over and over again. It becomes the never-ending quest for the perfect father (or mother), who does not exist.

The real challenge for a man who has not received his father's blessing is to separate his father's limitations from his own sense of worth. This is a jazzy way of saying you learn not to take other people's humanness personally. Easier said than done, I know. For many who carry this type of wound, a funny thing happens in these encounters with fathers and would-be father figures. That part of a man which is stuck as a little boy is engaged. All the emotions and thoughts related to a boy looking for his father's approval are conjured up again. When the man walks away feeling the same old paternal rejection, even if others pat him on the back and say, "You're a good man," he can't take those compliments to heart. This is because his ultimate authority on manliness—his father—doesn't approve of him. A man who has suffered this way often erects a protective wall around his heart that even healthy, loving care can't breach.

## The Two Fathers

There are two sets of fathers that need to be dealt with: the shadow father and the real father. The real father is different from the shadow father in terms of both time and perception. The shadow father is an old picture frozen in time from the formative years. They do not age; they stay the same and carry many of the same distressing or menacing characteristics from the past. The shadow father is a distorted and incomplete perception of who this person actually is in the real world. When the shadow father dominates the psyche, a man regresses back to being a boy with feelings of hopelessness and powerlessness. In these moments, a man loses touch with his own power. He fails to realize he is an adult now and has more influence to bring about a different outcome than he did in his childhood.

It may be hard to remember exactly what it was like to be a kid. To place yourself in the frame of reference of a small child is difficult to do. This is because almost everyone has progressed in many significant ways since then. We advance in the ways we deal with emotions and in our understanding of the complexities and nuances of others. Even our brains, which have not fully developed in childhood, have matured and allow us to see the world in all its complexity. In turn, this affects how we perceive the world and those in it.

But imagine going back to the days of childhood and recalling small elements of how primitive the world felt. Highly anticipated holidays or birthdays seemed as if they would never arrive; the concept of time seemed so incomprehensible. The intensity of your emotions was so strong, you felt like you might implode. Even the way you looked at people, as being either exclusively good or bad, was based on how they made you feel in the moment. When parents set limits like, "It's time for bed," they were not only "mean" but the worst people in the whole universe, until they morphed into loving parents again by the next morning.

The world of a child is very different from the one that most adults inhabit, and yet we sometimes revisit our childhood because parts of us are emotionally stuck there for many reasons. In some cases, we weren't cared for properly, or a disruptive trauma caused parts of our development to be arrested. Sometimes we revisit this primal world when old wounds get scratched. People may suddenly respond to a situation in a childlike manner, with over-the-top emotions. Those around us may ask, "What just happened? You were not yourself for a few moments." The honest answer is that we temporarily crossed over the bridge to the lost world of childhood that still resides within us.

You may have already guessed how the primal world of a child fits into our discussion here. Men who did not receive their father's blessing, for whatever reason, feel stuck. It is very hard to talk a child out of the emotions they feel, and for adult men, the same rule applies when they are mulling over the father wound from days gone by. It seems as though they don't use all of their adult abilities in those moments. They seem frozen in time, with an image of their father and themselves from way back then.

If a man grew up with an overbearing father, recalling his childhood may cause fear and trembling. The same man may live in apprehension as an adult, unable to shake the notion that he and his shadow father cannot do anything but repeat the same destructive exchange whenever they are in contact. The grip of the shadow image is strong, not allowing a man to move out of that simple realm of childlike experience; instead, he only sees the shadow father as an intimidating force that he has no power to influence. In this case, when he runs into the shadow father or someone like him, he regresses back to a childlike way of relating and feels emotionally overwhelmed. Someone who was a fully functioning adult a moment ago now becomes fear-struck and unable to use his adult skills. He may stumble over his words, feel powerless, or defer his authority because he is re-creating what he did when he was a child.

A man who lived in actual fear of his father while growing up once described to me the way his father would belittle him as a boy. He would essentially stand him in the corner and verbally attack him for his supposed shortcomings. These episodes seemed like they would go on forever, his father grimacing and getting so stirred up, he would spit as he yelled. The image of his overbearing father stayed in his mind even as an adult. Sometimes his father would call him on the phone when he was at work. The man once nervously dropped his pen under his desk during one of these calls. He held on to the phone as he crawled under his desk to retrieve his pen. And then a funny thing happened: the man noticed that he felt safer talking to his father under his desk. So he sat there and made it through the phone call. The man had discovered a very symbolic way of trying to buffer himself from the recollections of a verbally abusive past by constructing his own bomb shelter of sorts, helping him to weather the fear of an attack.

# Personalization-Pursuit Cycle

Personalizing the disappointments a man experienced with his caregivers and fixating on either shadow parent, like "Mom was supposed to supply this," or "Dad was supposed to do that," can send a male (boy or man) on a long-standing quest for the emotional treasure he felt he missed. He will seek to wrestle from the parent, shadow parent, or shadow parent stand-in what he believes is restitution for what he did not receive from them as a child. The phenomenon is called "personalization-pursuit cycle." Some men get hooked on chasing these images in whatever manifestation they appear, and it activates an archaic longing to capture what they never had. This drives some men to fits of rage, sadness, and despair. They know that at some level there is something very important at stake, but they dare not put it into words.

But now we know what it is that he is struggling with: it involves his core worth as a man, his value and lovability. When parents don't deliver needed care, a man will personalize the shortcomings, blaming himself for not being lovable (smart, good, etc.) enough. This will result in a never-ending pursuit of a person who can symbolically set him free. The major flaw in this logic is that the shadow parent(s) do not have the goods to deliver— that's how they earned the shadow image status in the first place. Many men bang their head against the wall trying to extract something from someone who does not have it to give. As we will see in the next chapter, men have to break the personalization-pursuit cycle to be set free from shadow parents. This involves turning to people who really *can* deliver and not chasing those who are unable.

There is one other similar issue to consider. Because the man has set up the personalize-pursuit dynamic, he will be inclined to pursue those that resemble shadow parent(s). These shadow parent stand-ins can include romantic partners, friends, bosses, or colleagues. People bearing a psychological resemblance to the shadow parents act as bait for his unresolved issues. He will feel drawn to these people, often at an unconscious level, stirring up a mixed array of reactions like hope, excitement, anger, and guardedness. After all, being faced with another encounter with a shadow parent specter and the possibility of feeling set free—or worse, being disappointed all over again—brings up a jumbled bag of reactions. He is primed to react to these shadow parent stand-ins, even if it is not in his best interests.

In the personalization-pursuit cycle, a man will try to fulfill unresolved needs from the past with a person who psychologically resembles his shadow parents. If a father was rejecting, a man might repeat a similar need for approval in interactions with other disapproving males. What complicates matters is when the unresolved need is stirred up in a relationship, but the target of pursuit doesn't match the original shadow parent in outer appearance or even gender. For instance the man mentioned earlier who has the legacy of a father wound may choose a wife who feels rejecting. It may seem ridiculous to him that he is in fact still carrying out (with his wife) the personalization-pursuit cycle from his father/son relationship. "But how can that be?" he may ask. "She is a woman and I am not gay or anything . . ." At the heart of this never-ending pursuit is the need to procure emotional nurturance from the shadow parent who rejected him, and that dynamic can play out in either gender, with straight or gay men. While the outer appearance can heighten shadow parent reactions, it is the emotional similarity that hooks people.

The mistaken notion that the personalization-pursuit cycle can only be played out with the exact carbon copy of the original shadow parent also sets up other stereotypes that involve who can help heal old wounds. This includes notions like a male can only find help with healing the father wound with another male or the mother wound with a female. In these cases, people may turn away from what could have been the deeper spirit of what was needed and longed for all along, because at first blush it didn't match the prepackaged version they hoped for. In my practice, both men and women who are contemplating their psychological legacies have said to me in frustration, "But how can you help me? You're a man." They believe that because I do not resemble the shadow parent on the surface level, I can offer no help. Many come to realize that it is not the outer appearance (the gender) that matters most, but rather the individual's capacity for deep emotional nurturance that allows healing to occur.

## Transforming the Shadow Father into the Real Father

It may be evident, but it is vitally important for a man to move the father out of the realm of shadows. A man does this by getting to know the second father—the one who is three-dimensional and fully formed—the *real father*. It may be hard to imagine that he is a real person beyond his role as parent. It is no small task to see his father in a more realistic light, free from perceptual distortions.

In the best healing situations, a man learns to place his now-adult eyes on the shadow father, transforming him into his real father. He tightens his focus on the once-distorted perceptions of the past and is now able to see his real father more clearly. This allows for a more complex understanding of who his caregiver is—an actual person in the real world with his own set of hopes, dreams, frustrations, hurts, and limitations. With this new realization, the journey from the shadow realm has begun, as a man liberates himself from the childlike perceptions that kept him bound.

This new access to information based in understanding and compassion redraws the image of the formerly disruptive shadow parent. He sees the real father age, notes his frailties, and can see him as less of a toxic force than how he remembered him from childhood. A man doing this type of shadow parent work can get to know and approach his father in ways that lead to healing and restoration for his heart and psyche. We will look more closely at making peace with the shadow parents in the next chapter.

# Mother/Son Relationship

You recall from the beginning of this chapter that the Industrial Revolution led to the divided spheres of work and home in society: the father was in charge of the world of work outside the home, and the mother was responsible for the duties within. This arrangement created built-in cultural expectations about what each parent traditionally contributed to the psychological development and welfare of their children. With boys, the father was in charge of goals and ambitions, teaching his boy how to be a man by helping him to master the roles of provider, protector, and progenitor in the world. The mother, by contrast, was symbolically associated with hearth and home. She was mistress of the realm of tender feelings, and her tutelage involved helping the boy emotionally connect with others. Mom would also provide a soft place to fall after a hard day's work at being a man. Sometimes she would even buffer those hard expectations, acting as intermediary between father and son.

The theory that a father helps a boy go out into the world of work and the mother is the ultimate source of tenderness is for some just a well-worn stereotype. As we know, there are situations where single moms (or dads) are forced to fill the sometimes-overwhelming roles and expectations of both parents. Each family has its own signature style regarding how these needs are met, to what degree, and by which parent. For instance, sometimes the father is the source of emotional affection, and sometimes the mother is better able to give instruction.

Today's men are sometimes in a quandary about changing gender roles and expectations, which are not delineated as well as the model of the past. To some extent, there is still a cultural expectation that moms are the ones who supply tenderness; many men sign on to this belief, and it affects them deeply. If their mom was not a source of tenderness, they wonder if she was the exception to the rule. That is, just like not receiving the father's approval, they wonder if mom's lack of warmth was a sign that they were not worthy of her love. After all, if a mother does not love her son, who will?

This wondering can become part of a man's psyche, often at an unconscious level. It can affect how a man sees himself and his relationships with others. It may take the form of wondering if women can be trusted for emotional support, or at the deepest level, if a woman can truly love him for who he is, warts and all. Men may think that perhaps they need to sweeten the deal through money, jewelry, or pheromone-laden cologne, like a Darwinian ape trying to secure the affections of women. It may be hard to accept that what they bring to the negotiation table beyond their personal essence could possibly be enough.

It is at this level that the fear of the feminine and the roots of misogyny are found. After all, from his perspective, mom (and perhaps the ensuing line of women) came up short on some important counts, and that leaves him in search of answers, or worse, revenge. As one of the commandments suggests, "If you don't please your mother, you must marry someone like her." A man will often unwittingly go in search of a potential romantic partner to put this old scenario to the test again, hoping that this time the outcome will be different. Perhaps he can find someone to love him just for him. This is serious stuff. A man needs to find out if this business is true; can he really count on a woman to value and love him for who he is?

Yet one of the binds women find themselves in is that while the societal stereotypes suggest that the ability to engender tender feelings (often referred to as the maternal instinct) is an innate part of being a woman, in reality there is a lot of variability within this dimension. Not all women are comfortable in the role of nurturer, and as female clients and friends have confessed to me, this is very troubling to them. There is a cultural expectation that all women meet at least the minimum standard as a nurturer, and when they don't, it is taken as a marker that they are less of a woman. Women often feel uncomfortable about not doing this part of motherhood (or partnerhood) better, and men often personalize the results, misinterpreting the women's lack of nurturing as a referendum on their worth as a man. In the end, both men and women are affected.

This is when the shadow mother, who boys and men simultaneously long for and fear, enters into their psyches. She can be a scary, magical creature who has the power to mend a broken portion of the heart, but she can also cast a spell that could rip the still-pumping organ from his chest. The challenge is to humanize this shadowed image; otherwise, love and fear will always walk hand in hand, dictating the tenor of the mother/son relationship *as well as romantic relationships.*

## ▶ Toolbox Tip: Personalization-Pursuit Cycle and the Mother Wound

One of the best movie examples of the legacy of the mother wound is the Academy Award–wining movie *Ordinary People*. Mary Tyler Moore plays a bereaved parent who lost her oldest son in a boating accident. Her surviving son, an adolescent boy named Conrad (or "Con," played by Timothy Hutton), cannot understand why his mother is so cold to him. His eventual conclusion is that she does not love him. This affects him deeply; he subsequently tries winning her approval and acceptance in an intense version of the personalization-pursuit cycle. This includes attempting to follow in his dead brother's footsteps by being on the swim team, making good grades, and even initiating hugs (though with no reciprocal response from his mother).

The internal pressure mounts to such a degree that Con attempts suicide. It is only after an intense period of therapy that he begins to reexamine his shadow parent and sees that she has limitations. Con comes to realize that it was difficult for his mother to show affection in the first place, but losing her other son completely shut her down emotionally. He begins to step away from the personalization-pursuit cycle by seeing the shadow mother in a different light, one marked by understanding and compassion. While it is still painful to miss out on that mother/son connection, it becomes more tolerable for him when he realizes that he is not to blame or "unlovable."

## THE LEGACY OF THE MOTHER WOUND
## IN ROMANTIC RELATIONSHIPS

One of the legacies of the mother wound involves the fantasy that a romantic partner will make up for all the emotional needs left unfulfilled. This can cause serious relationship issues. A partner who has an understanding of the mother wound in a man's life and the problems it can cause can significantly impact the relationship in positive ways.

Traditionally, it has been thought that the first relationship with a woman (Mom) supplies the model for what men expect of adult relationships with romantic partners (in reality, both parents contribute). Men may shy away from their male friends as a source of emotional support and instead envision their romantic partner as the person who will take care of a significant portion, if not all, of those types of needs.

There are a number of problems with this approach. First, this type of arrangement is innately burdensome to the romantic relationship. If we follow the stereotypical trajectory of a passionate connection, a man will at some point begin revealing more of who he is. When he begins to put away the cool poise and the bravado, he indicates to his partner he is ready for more of an honest and authentic relationship—a definite sign that feelings are deepening.

Most partners on the other side of this equation, if interested, will take this as a positive step. "Great," she thinks, "he is starting to open up to me." We all have public and private selves, those faces we show the world and those we only reveal to our innermost circle. We only show our private selves when there is a sense of emotional intimacy. However, this arrangement can get off-kilter when the man's partner has a well-developed social network that has access to her private side, and he only has her.

At first, she may feel flattered he has chosen her for this exclusive privilege. It is like he turns off the force field that surrounds the secret shoe box and she is the only other person who knows the secret code. It is all the more special if she is aware of the many risks and potential man-barriers connected to the commandments that her partner is hurdling by opening himself up to her. But this initial shine can lose some of its luster if he relies on her too much. One person cannot carry the entire intimacy load of the relationship, and this intensifies when the man in question has a significant legacy related to the commandments and the mother wound.

There is a strong potential for the personalization-pursuit dynamic to reactivate old shadow parent wounds, and this has a tendency to intensify the man's neediness, which in turn impacts both partners. He feels neglected, and she feels overburdened. The legacy of the mother wound comes alive in these situations. When the stress level becomes too much, some romantic partners begin to act out, feel put upon, and sometimes become more emotionally distant. This can take various forms, like setting up "play dates" for the man in hopes that he can find some additional support elsewhere, avoiding phone calls in anticipation of another needy conversation, or turning "date night" into double date night to inject fresh conversation and some needed space.

The degree of his unmet needs will dictate the amount of clarity with which he can seek emotional support outside of the romantic relationship. If he never experienced the safety of a nurturing relationship in the first place, then lingering hopes of finding a single source to meet all his needs will no doubt resurface. If the woman's knee-jerk reaction is to pull away, some men will experience this as eerily similar to the emotional rejection of the past when his mother was unable to fulfill his emotional needs. From the perspective of the boy frozen inside of the man, he sees his mother and those like her in a less-than-favorable light when he believes they are withholding what he so desperately needs.

If his partner is not privy to the painful legacy of his shadow mother, she will not understand the depth of what is being conveyed when he says, "But I do not want new friends, I just need you!" As he makes these remarks, you may catch a glimmer of the little boy bubbling up to the surface, unable to separate your need for breathing room from the painful legacy of his shadow mother's rejection.

There is a real danger that a romantic partner and shadow parent will become fused together in the psyche at this point. It can become the basis for stalkers in romantic relationships that ended badly or the painful pining of a lost love well past the relationship's expiration date. If the relationship continues, a shift in how the partners relate can occur; the man may become increasingly more like a boy. When this happens, there is more at stake than just getting your attention and emotional support. The personalization-pursuit cycle becomes fully engaged, a telltale marker that previous efforts from you are not enough for him. He will begin making demands that are even more unreasonable. He may not want to be separated from your side at parties where he once was charming and independent, or he may seem like he has been slighted to the extreme when you make mention that another man is "cute." Many women scratch their heads at this point and wonder, "Where has my man gone? It seems like he has been replaced by a demanding little boy!" Romantic partners envision the future of the relationship with some trepidation.

However, there is hope for the person who confuses the shadow parent and the romantic interest, even in a long-term relationship. Often it takes a period of "relationship safety" where a romantic partner shows there is a natural ebb and flow to relationships in day-to-day interactions. The man may begin to realize at an emotionally deep level that his partner's need for space is not equal to abandonment. One of the key things to remember in moments when the little boy resurfaces is that he is not grounded emotionally; he is under the influence of the shadow parent legacy. It is necessary to attune yourself to the remnants of the mother wound while simultaneously encouraging him to move forward toward healing.

For some men, this can play out in various levels of intensity over an extended period of time. The mother wound may be aggravated when transitions occur, such as new jobs, going back to school, relocation, pregnancies, and so on. These new situations, which introduce new forces, people, and places, can have an impact on a man's emotional lifeline. Jealousy, envy, territoriality, sulking, angry withdrawal, and more demands are common reactions in these situations. The little boy inside feels threatened, and a wise partner will reassure his partner, which helps him return to his former man stance.

## RELATIONSHIP RED ZONE:
### An Imbalance of Power

A problem infused with the shadow mother/significant other dilemma creates an imbalance of power in the romantic relationship. A man stuck in the personalization-pursuit cycle may feel like too much is at stake for maintaining a firm stance when needed; consequently, his erosion of power begins. After all, he does not want to lose his sole support, so he does what he must to avoid this at any cost. This can lead to all manner of problems, such as a wishy-washy attitude, acting conveniently unaware of his own emotions or needs so as not to come into conflict with yours, and a loss of respect for himself as a man. While sitcoms may suggest that women want a somewhat dim romantic partner who caves to her every whim, those who are in this situation soon lose either respect or interest in a male partner who is not his own man.

## ▶ Toolbox Tip: Mother Wound Discussion Points

Just as we discussed some of the identifiable aspects of the father wound, below are discussion questions that may lead to important conversations about the legacy of the maternal wound and its potential effect on romantic relationships. Discussing these questions with your partner may lead to significant healing in this area.

1. Does his relationship with his romantic partner account for nearly all his emotional support?

2. Is he uncomfortable turning to his other friends when discussing "sensitive issues" such as emotions?

3. Is his romantic partner the only person who really sees his most private face?

4. Does he struggle with the idea that his mother was not able to be there for him when he needed her emotionally?

5. Does he believe that his romantic partner should make up for needs that were not met when he was growing up?

6. Does he feel like he must concede to his romantic partner's wishes because, when it comes down to it, she really is the only person he has got?

7. Does he believe that people always leave unless he keeps them happy?

8. Does he feel like he has a hole deep inside that cannot be filled?

9. Do addictive behaviors like porn, gambling, and drinking give him momentary relief from the intense emotions he feels?

10. Is he afraid to let people know how needy he is?

# Conclusion

This chapter addressed the emotional remnants of the shadow parents that many men carry to some degree. We discussed how the Industrial Revolution caused delineation between men's work and women's work. In this model, the father supplies direction for his son, guiding him in his goals and ambitions and teaching him "how to be a man." The mother is responsible for the world of the home, including what it takes to be successful at the tasks of relational work, which is governed by the tender aspects of emotions. Psychologically speaking, these differing experiences come to represent a man's perceived sense of value and lovability.

When parents fail to give a boy what he psychologically needs, "shadow parents" can take up residence in a man's psyche. The commandments that related to parental wounds speak of these painful legacies where men wonder about their inherent worth. Though I have discussed the father and mother wounds based on traditional expectations and roles for simplicity's sake, the truth is that either parent can affect a man in the areas of worth and lovability. For most men, the emotional prerequisites for growing up healthy and happy in the areas of work and love are *not* linked to fulfilling the stereotypical notions of manhood. Having a good life is not about following someone else's model, but rather involves carving out one's own signature way of living. To live an authentic life, men will have women (moms, sisters, girlfriends, and wives) who shape their sense of masculinity in significant ways; likewise, men will be nurtured by other men (dad, brother, best friend, etc). Neither gender has a monopoly on the ability to supply or receive these types of experiences, regardless of societal stereotypes.

Until recently, psychology textbooks still divided the gender world neatly and consistently into separate spheres, but fortunately, that perspective has begun to change. Today's moms and dads will not necessarily follow the old formula based on traditional gender-based responsibilities. Gender does not preclude the ability to offer the emotional nutrients involved in helping someone develop his (or her) sense of value or lovability. Many children who are raised by single moms or dads are healthy, happy children with strong self-images.

In the next chapter we will learn how to make peace with the shadow parent images, which will lead to a more fulfilled life. Imagine not having to carry around all the baggage from childhood and being able to function on a more adult level in the areas of work and love. Making peace with the shadow parents will also assure that you don't pass the legacy on to your children or romantic partner.

# CHAPTER CUES

1. Contemporary gender stereotypes are based on misconceptions regarding the division of the spheres of responsibility in parenting into men's work and women's work.

2. While the gap has closed in terms of really understanding what men and women are capable of, there is still a biased notion about men being solely responsible for turning a boy into a man or women solely supplying emotional nurturance.

3. There are two sets of parents: the real parents and the shadow parents.

4. Shadow parents exist in a frozen state of mind where they are two-dimensional, seen through the eyes of a child. This can lead to trouble functioning in the adult world of responsibilities.

5. Men often lose touch with their adult skills and instead regress to childlike ways of functioning because of lingering shadow parents.

6. When shadow parent images or stand-ins are encountered, they usually result in a mixed set of reactions, such as hope, fear, anger, or guardedness.

7. Those fully under the sway of inner shadow parent images look in the wrong places and relationships to meet unmet needs from childhood.

8. A personalization-pursuit cycle governs many men's lives.

9. The ability to change a shadow parent into a real parent is accomplished through seeing him or her with adult eyes.

10. In order to break the personalization-pursuit cycle men have to think outside the box and break the commandments to be set free.

# 8

# Making Peace with the Shadow Parents

In the previous chapter, we learned that a shadow parent is an incomplete and somewhat skewed view of a caregiver, formed and frozen in time from the incomplete perspective of a child. A shadow parent image is created from fragmented pictures of caregivers that represent disappointing experiences from the past. They are the remembered snapshots of emotional letdowns, and, feeling undervalued or abandoned. Some of these are the results of the "normal difficulties" we all face in growing up, trying to obtain a more mature perspective of caregivers and ourselves. Other images reflect particularly harsh circumstances that left substantial damage.

Shadow parent images are carried around in our psyches and hearts. Sometimes they lie dormant, and other times they spring to life. When they make their presence known, shadow parent images elicit strong primal emotions that can be overwhelming. Grown adults can feel as though they have turned back the hands of time, instantly returning to childhood. When this occurs, adults feel stripped of their mature skills and talents. They stand powerless in the presence of the shadow parent. When shadow parent images are embedded in the psyche, they need to be brought into the light and then set to rest, or the legacy of suffering continues.

Making peace with the parental shadows is hard work; it can be a long and difficult journey. I am always amazed by self-help infomercials that claim they can change your life in seven days through listening to subliminal tapes that help you find the secret to eternal peace or weekend seminars that can make all relationship woes magically disappear! A colleague of mine once asked me if I would be willing to chip in on a videotape that claimed the same epic, life-changing potential for just "three easy payments of $99.95." The TV guru guaranteed easy and painless transformation. I will admit that it sounded pretty tempting. While I am sad to report that no one has stumbled onto the easy path to peace and contentment, we can receive healing in significant ways as we look at the important relationships that have impacted us most throughout our lives.

While there are many important people in a man's life, the parental relationships supersede all others, because they helped form his core personality and perspective on the world and others. The notion that these connections from the past still carry such importance does not always sit well; as one man asked me, "Why do I have to talk about the past? After all, it's in the past." Issues are only truly in the past when they no longer have power over us. As we have seen, the Ten Commandments of Growing Up Male are far-reaching and can have an effect on a person in ways he may not always be aware; he just knows that in secret moments, old familiar hurts arise, causing problems in the areas of work and love.

Uncovering the root of these troubles and then putting them to rest is not easily done. Often the path to a more peaceful life has to be walked over and over again until the obstacles on the road can be removed. This pursuit of healing in the areas that are damaged or in need of care when properly attended to can produce unexpected flowers of wisdom and compassion. This chapter provides an overview of some of the work your partner, family member, or friend may need to go through on this journey. While he is ultimately the one who must do these tasks, it is important that you be aware of what to expect, and while this is primarily for the men in your life, you may find many of the same approaches useful in your own quest for inner peace. Maybe you and your man can walk this road together.

# An Incomplete Peace

A man makes peace with his shadow parents for himself and those he loves, but many men get hung up on the idea that making this type of effort is really just another concession to a parent who was abusive or neglectful emotionally and/or physically. He may think, "I don't want to do this; it only means they still have power over what I do, think, or feel." In many cases the shadow parent versions still *do* have power over his present life whether he recognizes it or not. Making peace with his shadow parents places power back into the man's hands so he can choose how to live and be his own person.

In the clinical setting, people who are working on putting aspects of their shadow parent(s) to rest have difficulty assessing where they are in this process. Sometimes a person says he has completed this important work, but he'll say it with angry resolve. His solution might be that he wants nothing more to do with his caregivers. Many people mistakenly interpret this as being done with the shadow parent work; they believe if they ignore or shut out the problem, they have found "peace." In reality, these people are still invested, and consequently they are still connected to the legacy of the past. They have just learned to temporarily cut off or compartmentalize the longing, anger, or hurt.

I had a student once who wanted to do men's research with me because he wanted to prove "how screwed up men are." I nearly did a double take when listening to his reasoning for how he would spend the next few years doing research. The student later revealed to me that his father had ruined his and his family's life because of, among other things, his detached emotional manner. He wanted to confirm that being like his father was unhealthy and even pathological. I could only imagine the result of this student's fantasy. On the day of completion, he could present his research paper to his father and unequivocally prove the point that their encounters were hurtful. While this student stated he wanted nothing more from his father, it was apparent that he was still very invested in the shadow parent from the past; after all, his shadow father was still dictating his behavior. Many men are still trying to settle scores from the past but don't realize they are doing so.

The more difficult path of finding peace with shadow parents involves a different process: it requires emotionally disengaging from anger and hurt, as well as letting go of the desire for old wishes to come true. Through grief and eventual acceptance, people can come to terms with the past, and a sense of peace can replace the intense feelings of emptiness, disappointment, and sadness. This approach breaks the ties to old experiences that keep men from being free and gives them the opportunity to have more control in their lives now. It literally allows them to be their own men.

It also allows for a different quality of connection with caregivers; the relationship is brought to a more adult level where real individuals are engaged in relating to each other, and the shadowy remnants of the past have less power to intrude into conversations. Much of the distortion of the past acts as a barrier for present interactions, whether with real parents, shadow parents, or shadow parent stand-ins. When men make peace with the shadow images, they see themselves and their parents in a new light marked by compassion for the human frailty we all carry.

## ▶ Toolbox Tip: Toxic Parents

As someone trying to support a man who has shadow parent issues, you may initially encounter some resistance; he may be hesitant to take the steps to heal those types of relationships. Some men will react skeptically to the idea of coming to peace with their shadow parents and ask, "Does this mean I have to forgive all that has happened? Do I have to be friendly with this person after all they put me through?" The short answer is that men have to at least make peace with the shadow parents, but extending that work to the real parent can often help. There are extreme situations where continued interaction with real parents is so toxic that healing the relationship becomes impossible. This may be the case when they are chronically impaired, using drugs and/or alcohol, or engaging in physical violence. Until those situations are different, work with the actual parent is not possible. But this does not preclude men from coming to terms with the shadow parents, the ones who reside within. He cannot change the real people his parents are, but he can learn how to control and dispel the lingering shadow images he has unintentionally created.

# Rites of Transformation

Sometimes it is useful to look beyond psychology to find help for making peace with one's inner world. In his book *Rites of Passage* (1909), anthropologist Arnold van Gennep defines a *rite* as that "which accompanies every change of place, state, social position, and age." Rites are the tangible steps or guidelines that help a person through a transformation. Rites provide a much-needed structure in a chaotic and messy time. In most cases, rites include a ceremony, spoken words, and/or symbols or symbolic acts that reflect actual change. What does this have to do with shadow parent work? One of the most difficult transformations in life involves changing a person's inner world. Shadow parents reside within the heart and mind. If they stay in their current state, they evoke pain and cause a man to stumble on his life path. Our hope is that shadow parents can be transformed, resulting in a sense of peace for the person who has carried them. To help with this transformation or any like it, this complicated process needs order and structure.

## ▶ Toolbox Tip: Different Rites of Transformation

Below is a list of different types of rites of transformation and examples for each. As you can see, they occur at all levels of society, both at the personal and cultural level. Some are contemporary and easily recognized while others are a part of the older cultural backdrop.

1. Individual rites: such as puberty rites, when a boy emotionally or physically becomes a man
2. Religious rites: baptism, when one enters the faith
3. Ceremonial rites: marriages, when two people join as one
4. Societal rites: fertility or harvest rituals marking the beginning or ending of the growing season
5. Political rites: inauguration of a president or coronation of a monarch

Van Gennep argued that all rites of transformation go through an ordered process that includes three phases: (1) the separation phase, (2) the liminal phase, and (3) the assimilation phase. The first phase, *separation*, consists of the individual detaching from the previous identity or status. In this phase, he literally separates from his old notion of who he is. Very often, a period of physical separation from the familiar world also accompanies this stage of change. In some cases, this involves a new designated physical space a person occupies or visits to denote in symbolic terms that he is making a break from the past and preparing for a new life. This is a ceremonial place for transformation.

The next phase is the *liminal* one. The individual occupies what anthropologist Victor Turner referred to as a place "betwixt and between" where one's former identity is released and the new identity slowly becomes fashioned. This phase is the most difficult one, often characterized by pain, confusion, and grief, but also, ultimately, by a deep sense of transformation. The old adage, "no pain, no gain" aptly applies here. The trials and tribulations that are encountered forge the new identity. Graduation from the liminal phase is accompanied by a symbolic act where the old self dies or is put to rest and the new person emerges. The actual rite can take many forms (as we will soon see), but there is something powerful about these symbolic acts that reflects the emergence of the new inner world of the individual.

Finally, when the "new" person has been cast, he reenters the world in the *assimilation* phase. Because the person has transformed, this phase focuses on knitting his new identity into his old world. This is not always an easy thing to do. After all, he is a different person now, and that includes assuming new rights and responsibilities. This also affects relationships with family and friends, some of whom may be wary about these new changes.

These phases of transformation can be of assistance in the peacemaking process with shadow parents. As I mentioned previously, one of the most difficult transformations anyone can undergo is altering his or her inner world; it is not as simple as rearranging the furniture in the living room. When the inner world begins to change, the whole person is affected: how they think, feel, act, and how they see the world, relationships, and themselves. In the midst of what can be a very chaotic time, the abiding structure of each of the phases that accompanies the rite of transformation (separation, liminal, and assimilation) will be a significant aid in this process. In the following sections, I will go into detail about the work that occurs during each phase as it applies to making peace with the shadow parents.

# Separation (Phase 1)

First, the individual makes the decision to separate from his prior way of seeing the shadow parents. This decision can occur for many reasons. He may experience feelings of dissatisfaction or dysfunction that lead him to finally say "enough" with the old way of perceiving or doing things. Sometimes the present methods used to negotiate the world of the shadow parents lead only to anger and frustration. Holiday visits always seem to pick up where they left off, reengaging the same heated arguments from previous years. After so many of these episodes, a man may conclude that this level of toxicity is too much to carry any longer.

A man may also start the separation process when he realizes that his parents are aging and they will not be around forever. The thought of them passing away may spur him on to gain some sense of peace before they die. Another common occurrence that may lead to the first phase of separation is when a man becomes a father and begins seeing the shadow parents from a different perspective. Maybe he discovers with some unease that he and his shadow father or mother have remarkably similar parenting styles. He may have a sobering moment when he realizes that avoiding passing on the same legacy to his children means making peace with the shadow parents he carries inside. Any or all of these reasons may cause a person to long to make things different. The essence of the separation phase is an attitude that embraces the readiness for transformation; often this is accompanied by an actual physical separation to a place where the hard work is done.

## The Separation Phase: Creating a Space for Change

In the original anthropological studies that van Gennep's book was based on, he noted that a symbolic ceremonial area was often incorporated into various rituals. Having this ritual space gave the rite a special meaning and significance. It broke from everyday activities and caused the individual(s) to assume a different frame of mind, focusing attention on his or her inner world. Depending on the culture and the time period, this ceremonial space might be a hut, a cave, a circle of standing stones, or a majestic cathedral. Adding to the atmosphere would be artifacts of special importance pertaining to the transformation that was to occur. These could include texts, pictures, or statues, all of which helped set the mood and focus on the rite that was to follow.

A parallel space can also be established for the work with shadow parents. An individual leaves his normal world in order to purposefully and mindfully step into this symbolic arena. The exact setting can vary: a quiet basement, study, a favorite spot out in the woods, or even a therapy office. All of these can become designated sites of transformation. Creating the right atmosphere helps him to engage in a way that might not normally be done. The "artifacts" can be as elaborate as the person feels is necessary: pictures of parents or of himself, a journal, music, or whatever else is helpful in establishing this space as a thoughtful, meditative place. Logistically speaking, it is also helpful to choose a time that creates a sense of privacy, such as when loved ones are away or after they have gone to bed, so this time will not be interrupted. After all, if one is to experience transformation of the inner world, it has to be mindfully sought and free from distractions. Many people have to fight their normal compulsion to multitask—sitting down in front of the TV to watch Monday night football and attempting to do the next round of shadow parent work probably won't produce the results you want.

## ▶ Toolbox Tip: Relationships as the Ultimate Safe Zone

Consider the aspects that give a space a healing atmosphere: symbolic elements, the appropriate time frame, and a singular focus. All of these help create a safe environment that is conducive to healing. A man can experience deep psychological benefits from the actual physical spaces where his shadow work begins; it can be like going to a primal cave where tough, raw emotions can be expressed safely. It is important for a man to have a firm support to lean on when he is feeling undone inside. The necessary grief work that accompanies shadow work can be overwhelming, so having a safe place to go is important.

A very pertinent parallel exists between the physical space described above and the special type of relationship we talk about throughout this book, where a significant other in a man's life provides a safe place for him to express himself, the good and the bad, within the relationship. Both of these spaces allow the same types of healing experiences to occur. True healing happens when your man can feel safe enough to let it all hang out in his relationship with you. Allowing him to feel grounded amid the chaos helps him on his road to healing. There will be times when he needs to retreat to his "cave" for his own private time to work things out, but ultimately, you are the key person who provides a safe zone amid the difficulties of the shadow work. Relationships are the contexts in which many of our emotional/psychological wounds occur, but they are also the key source of healing.

### ▶ Toolbox Tip: Activities in the Ritual Space

With the ritual space created, a man begins to find ways to access the inner world. Sometimes people will keep a journal, allowing them to write about specific episodes from the past that come to mind. Others might enter a meditative state of mind where they let their attention wander to the damaged areas in their hearts and psyches. Sometimes they talk into a tape recorder. For some it is helpful to write letters to parents to access old feelings. Men can even create art in this space, painting and drawing; whatever feels right to them and represents these old conflicts.

# Liminal (Phase 2)

Of all of the phases, the liminal one is the roughest. The word *limen* is actually Latin for "threshold," so in the liminal phase, a man is on the threshold of change. This is the phase where the hard work of transformation occurs. There are a number of myths and stories that address the disorienting quality of this type of transitional period. It is like your own personal twilight zone. Often this place is covered in a fog that does not allow for clear sight or direction. A person may feel enveloped by this shadow work, but simultaneously not know exactly how to do it or bring it to a close.

After enough of the psychological and emotional prep work has been done, the particular shadow parent issue reaches critical mass as old troubles are confronted, released, and/or transformed. Sometimes this involves letting go of old hopes and wishes that will never come true. Other times, it involves new, deeper insights into the person who bears the lifelong job title of caregiver. It includes developing empathy, compassion, and understanding for the more complete person beyond the shadow parent. These experiences, while difficult, ultimately purchase a sense of relief.

Liminal moments are transformations that involve a just-noticeable difference in the inner world. That is, there is not the expectation that the troubles with shadow parents are dealt with in one fell swoop, in a singular liminal moment. While Hollywood movies would suggest otherwise, real-life peacemaking involves a collection of liminal moments in which bits of change occur over time. People keep working with their shadow parents, and each little liminal moment sets the stage for another to occur until a sufficient amount of change takes place.

Sometimes people doing this work feel discouraged because after making some gains and earning a deeper sense of peace, they still have more work to do. This is a normal part of the process and should not be interpreted as "all that hard work has accomplished nothing." A different way to look at this is comparing it to learning any new type of skill: making peace also takes some fine-tuning.

## The Liminal Phase: Grief Work

You may be thinking, "Well, this chapter sounds nice, but how does a man really get to the place of peace with the shadow parent(s)?" In large part, he will come to a more balanced place through grief. Grief is a natural reaction when coming to terms with the frustrating and disappointing snapshots of the shadow parents he carries around in his heart and mind. Each of these firmly ensconced images represents a collection of experiences that occurred over time. These images have to be reexperienced and then grieved over; otherwise, a person stays bound to the past.

It is not just the painful memories that a man is dealing with when he considers his shadow parents, but the grief of unfulfilled expectations as well. While they may be too embarrassed to acknowledge it (sometimes even to themselves), some adult men still carry strong hopes and wishes for a different type of care—a care they wanted but never received from their parents.

Some may wish that they could have a mom who would praise their ambition more; others long for a father who could be more emotionally available, someone he could feel comfortable going to when times were tough. Hanging on to these past hopes and wishes does not help achieve peace, but instead generates a constant state of hunger and disappointment for how things could have been: "If only my parent could have given me what I needed; my life would be so different now. I would have been successful and happy." This thought process often causes a downward spiral of sadness or anger followed by blaming all the failures and letdowns in his life on the shadow parents; in effect, he holds his shadow parent(s) hostage for subsequent missteps. If he cannot wrestle these archaic needs from his real parents, then shadow parent stand-ins perpetuate the personalization-pursuit cycle we discussed in the previous chapter. This energy can morph into misplaced hope or even revenge fantasies that one day he'll be able to settle the score with his shadow parent or stand-in (a boss, teacher, therapist, romantic partner, etc.) who is eerily similar to how he remembers his caregivers. This path does not lead to freedom; instead, a man in this place has no peace and remains a prisoner to the shadow images he carries.

While a man cannot change the actual events of the past, he can revisit them in a way that allows for a sense of peace. To do this he will need certain tools to aid him along the way. For instance, I often tell both male and female clients that there are two kinds of strength. The first involves being able to hold painful emotions in check. This is the one most people usually associate with being strong; that is, the ability to keep emotional or physical pain under control. We definitely need this one if are going to make it in this world.

However, it is the second definition of strength that allows people to be set free from chronic emotional wounds and the prison of the past. This involves the mindful decision to face the pain head-on in order to let it go. This is a counterintuitive definition of strength, as it requires revealing and encountering our deepest vulnerabilities. This is about moving beyond the acceptance of these things, as in, "I realize logically there is nothing that can be done about the past," to a more visceral acceptance, where emotions are confronted and then set to rest. This journey does not come at an easy price, since old hurts and disappointments come back to life with this process; it's like taking a trip back in time and reliving them firsthand. But the choice to step directly into the pain, allowing a scarred wound of the past to reopen, allows the healing to begin.

## ▶ Toolbox Tip: Time Machine Fantasy

There is no miraculous time machine that allows people to alter the past and get shadow parent(s) to change the course of personal histories. Yet it is common for people to stubbornly hold on to this type of magical thinking in the most secret part of their hearts. The power and intensity of these old wishes and fantasies tells us something about the depth of hurt that occurred and also how early on in life it began to be felt. It parallels the magical thinking of a young child: if only they wish hard enough, the past can magically be erased or refashioned.

## ▶ Toolbox Tip: The Ransom Game

A stumbling block in the peacemaking process can occur when the shadow parents and the real parents are involved in a ransom game. For instance, some may think, "Well, I can give up on the past and forgive the shadow parents if my real father or mother is willing to do some of the things now that I needed back then." Taking this approach becomes a slippery slope. A person could place far too much energy into getting their parent to fulfill a never-ending checklist of requirements before peace is found. Sometimes this becomes a protracted battle that is played out repeatedly during holiday visits. He may leave with the same feelings of frustration because nothing ever changes—and this would be a correct conclusion, because he is essentially committing to holding his breath until his real parent alters his/her behavior. Too many sons turn blue in the face waiting for this to happen. Instead, the goal is to let go to find peace.

## The Liminal Phase: Good Grief

So, you may ask, "Are you telling my man to just go somewhere and weep or feel sad?" The answer is no, it is more than that. We probably all know people who have made sadness a part of their daily routine. For some, sorrow about old events, injuries, or emotional wounds may begin to feel like an old familiar friend—not a good one, but nonetheless a recognizable one. Without it, they wouldn't know how to act; it becomes a central way they construct the way they see the world, people, and themselves.

For people stuck in this place, there is a bittersweet melancholy about their hurt. A part of them wants to listen to sad songs or see movies that remind them of their own pain. Some will get drunk and revel in what happened and what could have been. They think at some level that nothing can be done about this misery other than to bear it. I am not suggesting that the man in your life follow this example when trying to find peace with the past. Instead, there is the choice to move into the pain with the goal of letting it go so he can move forward with his life. This is a purposeful sadness, and its goal is freedom from suffering. Many people go through this type of process en route to finding healing.

In the liminal phase of transformation, a man begins to mindfully wander into the primal forest of his inner world. It may turn into some surreal dream where he is flooded with emotionally charged recollections of past hurts: mental portraits of father/son outings that went wrong, sibling rivalries that evoke fears of unbalanced parental alliances, or his first substantial parental letdown. While painful, this is the emotional fuel that propels him through the journey of grief; it will lead to other memories and connections that begin to form the emotional and mental picture of the shadow parent(s).

As a man wanders through this twilight zone, he collects bits and pieces of his past, trying to reconstruct an accurate picture of how things were. Sometimes, siblings and friends are also asked to contribute their shared memories. This will eventually lead to a transformation as, bit by bit, the shadow parent takes a more three-dimensional form. What was once shady and somewhat frightening can take on a more solid appearance. What seemed like monsters carried around in the psyche are made human. When this begins to happen, it will have an impact not only on the inner realm, but on the outer world with real parents as well. As in many myths and legends about the liminal world, it is very helpful to have a sidekick, friend, or companion to help sort through the experiences in this otherworldly place. If you have your hiking boots on, maybe you can join him for a walk in the primal woods. "How was your day, dear?" you ask. "Slay any ogres today?"

### ▶ Toolbox Tip: Two Perspectives

A person finds peace with shadow parents through the integration of two divergent perspectives: a child's and an adult's. The child's perspective is what created the skewed picture of the shadow parent. While often leading to an unbalanced view of things, it can be helpful now to recall how things felt as a child, to engage with the emotional perception of parent/child interactions. By contrast, the adult perspective supplies a more mature set of eyes, allowing a more complex consideration of people and events.

Imagine a child who feels all the intensity of the primal world but doesn't know what to make of it, and then a caregiver steps in to repackage the events in a more manageable way. We have discussed the important role of a *repackager* in the context of a caregiver/child relationship earlier in the book (see Chapter 6). In a similar way, the childlike part of the psyche brings the emotionally laden picture of caregivers and the drama that surrounded them to the adult part of the mind with the hope of finding a clearer, more peaceful picture. The result is that the emotional energy of the child integrates with the more mature perspective of an adult. A person's emotional resources are thus steadied and energized.

## The Liminal Phase: Following the Thread to the MAP

For some men it is more difficult to plunge headlong into the world of grief; after all, this type of emotional exploration is counter to the commandments that tell a man to mask his emotions. Now he may have to train himself to be aware of when his everyday life provides openings to the painful legacy of the past. I will outline three steps, using the acronym MAP, which stands for Monitoring and Assessing (themes from the) Past. Each of these will give tangible guidance for how to find the shadow parent issues that need to be grieved.

The first step concerns Monitoring what is going on in the difficult and unsettled areas of one's life. Steps toward change begin by just observing. Sometimes, in an overenthusiastic fervor, people begin moving things around in their lives too quickly or taking drastic steps because of the pressure "to do something." This can lead to rash decisions they later regret, like leaving their wives, quitting their jobs, or gambling house deeds away at a blackjack table. While it may make some a little antsy, the first step really is to do nothing and get a clear picture of what is going on. This is referred to as establishing a "baseline." That is, before moving anything around in one's life situation, a clearer picture of what is going on now must be achieved. Then, as the underlying complexity becomes better known, a more focused and lasting solution can be sought. While Monitoring may seem like the "lazy man's" way toward change, it is anything but that. Taking note of subtle complexities takes real effort.

Assessing involves discerning the day-to-day fluctuations in his emotional intensity and behavioral reactions. This includes both happenings at home and work and involves discerning the daily ups and downs from those more chronic pains from the past that need to be healed. A good rule of thumb: issues that have a basis in past troubles will have a much greater emotional reactivity. They may seem to go from zero to sixty in a matter of seconds and involve intense versions of emotions such as anger, sadness, shame, and so on. Another telltale sign is if he is having trouble disengaging from the particular incident of the day: he cannot sleep, plays it over and over in his head, feels too revved up, or is too angry to let it go. This suggests he is struggling with an issue from his past. Later, when he has finally calmed down, another accurate gauge is discerning if he can admit that the actual event that occurred did not warrant such an intense reaction. There may be some head-scratching about why this sort of thing always pushes his buttons, but these types of situations may show that he is mired in unfinished business.

The last step, Past, involves examining how the intensity of reactions are related to particular themes from the past. This occurs by monitoring and assessing present situations at work or home for familiar issues from the past, usually involving shadow parents. The goal is to see how old conflicts are being re-created in the present day. Usually people emotionally pick up right where they left off from childhood; they just plug the new shadow parent stand-ins (boss, coworker, romantic partner, etc.) into the old slot formerly filled by the caregiver. They revisit old familiar conflicts when they try to get overbearing people to recognize their sense of individualism or have others nurture unmet needs or value their contributions.

These patterns of interaction become the "same song, different verse" for many people who are trying to find peace with the past. When a man revisits the familiar ground of disappointment and hurt due to a pattern from the past, it is at this point that he must ask himself, "Are these feelings and reactions in the present situation familiar to any old stuff from the past?" He may start to realize that his anger toward a boss at work is similar to his feelings toward his father.

He may begin to determine not only the level of intensity in his reactions to everyday events, but also the types of things (or themes) that provoke him. He can begin developing a profile of hot-button topics that are sure to evoke a strong reaction. For instance, does the feeling of being reprimanded or undervalued bring more than its share of emotional conflict to the surface? Are there certain people, like an older man or woman, who seem to generate these reactions, and, if so, under what circumstances? He may have to do a little detective work to uncover the areas that are vulnerable to intense reactions.

The key to moving beyond what happened today may be to focus more on the related incidents that occurred in the past. Eventually, he will recognize that the sadness or disappointment that originated with the shadow parent is being brought into his present life. On closer examination, he may think, "This is exactly how I felt when I was a kid, and my shadow mother (or father) acted in a similar way."

Usually there are specific stories that go along with uncovering these feelings, and it helps to tell them. A good way to do this is through "free association"; that is, a person does not block the thoughts and feelings that suddenly spring to mind even if at first it seems as though they are far-reaching or disconnected from the current issue. People often access their episodic memory from various entry points of a story or recollection. Sometimes these are straightforward like, "I remember when . . . " while other times, feelings that are too powerful to bear can appear in more symbolic form, through dreams or tucked away safely by only recalling small details. These types of memories are often phrased like, "Gee, I do not know if this has anything to do with what we are talking about, but I remember when I was a kid . . ." If your man has gotten to this place, he is capable of an important insight: old troubles are a barrier in his present life and relationships. The good news is this can be fixed. The work that occurs between the shadow and real parent can be some of the most difficult and yet most rewarding that can occur in the liminal phase. The goal is to have the parent who resides within match the one who lives in the real world. When gains are made in one realm, it often has a direct effect on the other.

By continuing to do this exercise, he is constructing a thematic map of his inner world. In this process, he will uncover themes from the past that provoke strong reactions in the present. This will help him identify when the shadow parent images are operative. By approaching themes from both past and present perspectives, a clearer idea of issues and images that need to be squared away is reached.

## ▶ Toolbox Tip: Follow the MAP for Grief

These are tangible ways a man can find his approach into shadow parent grief. The MAP acronym below gives a summary for the work described above.

## MAP

**M** = Monitoring one's life (initially, without making change)

**A** = Assessing the intensity of emotional reactions, looking for hot–button areas

**P** = Past themes help construct an internal map of how shadow parent(s) relate to current happenings

## The Liminal Phase: Engaging the Real Parents

In the best-case scenarios, real parents are willing and able to engage men in this process of making peace with the past. There certainly will be lots of variation on this dimension. Defensiveness about the past, as well as declining mental abilities, are chief troublemakers on this journey. Those who are willing and present have their own peace to make with the past as well. I have certainly heard my share of stories from aging parents who sometimes, unbeknownst to their adult children, really want to set these things right. The feeling that they let their kids down weighs heavily on them. In the best situations, this type of work can lead to mutual healing for both parties. Sometimes, through much work, both parents and children can gain an understanding of the past.

At some point, most people ask "Why? Why didn't my caregiver(s) do a better job?" I do believe that, in most situations, caregivers do the best they can. Even in rather extreme situations involving emotional or physical abuse, I believe most parents wish they could have done better. Even this wish, however, does not always permit them to openly admit where they failed. Often parents personalize their shortcomings as caregivers as much as children personalize being on the short end of the stick in terms of care. It does not excuse this terribly damaging behavior; it just speaks to the caregivers' own limitations.

This "caregivers did the best they could" explanation may be hard for some to accept, especially if there is still anger and resentment from these painful experiences from the past. A person may remember trying to make sense of all the hurt that occurred. What kids often do in these disappointing situations is try to find some reason for their parent's inability to take better care of them. Because kids live in a different world in terms of cognitive and emotional capabilities, they muster up the best explanation they can based on their limited skills and experience. Often they come to the conclusion that their parents could do better, but for some reason—like being lazy or mean—they just would not.

Another explanation children may come up with is one of self-blame: "I know my parents want to give me good care, but they cannot because I am a rotten kid; if I can become a better kid they will see this and take care of me." The child uses this coping skill to preserve hope that goodness really does exist in the world, and if they hang on tight or work hard enough, they will finally experience the love and care they need. It is a survival skill that makes the child feel like they have some control.

All of these explanations can still haunt children when they become adults. They wrestle with the "whys" of not receiving better care. For instance, some adults are driven to prove their worth to their caregivers through achievements or success because of the way they understand their bargain. If they are just better people, they will get someone to love them. Some people hold their parents and other "lazy underachievers" in contempt but not completely realize why. What people fail to do when they operate from these explanations is move beyond the childlike realm where they attempted to explain away the hurtful situation. These accounts were the best a child could assemble given their limitations. There is a point as adults where we need to move beyond these interpretations that keep us bound to the past. What can help a person do this is to move beyond seeing caregivers solely and exclusively as parents.

As kids, we naturally see our parents as fairly two-dimensional. They only exist to serve our needs. We do not realize they are people with their own needs and wants—before and after they became our caregivers. Our explanation for our caregivers' shortcomings can carry the same lack of sophistication and naïveté. In order to turn a shadow parent into a multidimensional person, one has to develop a sense for who this person is apart from their role as caregiver.

A way of establishing a different, more adult relationship is to find out about them as individuals—their hopes and dreams, how it was for them to grow up, what their parents were like, the struggles they faced. Our caregivers may be a little sheepish at first in discussing these matters. After all, they are used to having the shoe on the other foot and trying to attend to us. But most people like talking about themselves to someone who is sincerely interested.

While this may be a fact-finding mission, it also establishes a new precedent for how you will relate together. You are inviting them to be real people, not two-dimensional cutouts from the past. The desired outcome of this kind of new interaction is to enrich the connection with parents in the hope that this will also have an impact on the shadow versions.

The nature of my relationship with my mom shifted over the last ten years of her life. When I visited and we had a few quiet minutes together, I would ask questions about the pictures of family she had on the walls or her memories of growing up. Sometimes I found out new things about her or relatives that were interesting, while other times I heard some painful stories that helped me to understand more about how my mother struggled. Once, to my surprise, she told me about her hopes and dreams of graduating from college and becoming a counselor, and how disappointed she felt because her family didn't see the value in sending "a farm girl to college." She also told me stories of feeling like she could never fill the void that was created when her older brother tragically died as a child. These experiences were a few of the many that slowly began changing the shadow version of my mother into a more real person, adding new dimensions that included endearing vulnerability and compassion.

This type of shadow parent work begins to have an impact on childlike expectations and leftover hurts. While trying to understand the past and place it into a new perspective, there is also the shedding of misplaced hope that parents (real or shadow) will finally come through on things. Instead, there is a choice to visit for connection's sake, and perhaps to make another pass at finding more peace. We may even say to ourselves, "I will not expect from my caregivers the things they cannot give. They were not able to give what I needed when I was a kid and they're not able to do it now. I will not hold them accountable for that any longer."

When we can say this and feel it deep in our core, we have come through to the other side of sadness and grief. There is the realization and acceptance that these necessary losses cannot be changed. This is a step toward being set free. What we are really doing is not only forgiving our parents for their human frailties, we are also coming to terms with our own. After all, a part of the shadow parent resides within us. No doubt we carry some of their dispositions and characteristics. To forgive the parent is in a way making peace with some part of ourselves with which we are not entirely at ease. This realization may also spur on the balanced decision to say, "Certain shadow parent behaviors that I have do not suit me any longer. I will choose to be different now." Coming to this realization may lead to changes in child-rearing practices or how one treats themselves and others. All these shifts lead to the removal of angry and sad feelings about the parent.

For most of us, this is serious stuff that has caused loads of pain. When we are able to disengage and heal that portion of ourselves, we can begin to see the parent in a different light. When parents do what they have always done—interrupt, or change the topic when it gets too emotional, seem unable to appreciate what we do, or always need to add their two cents—it does not have to initiate the old rage or disappointment. Rather, we can approach this in a more even manner and reframe these experiences as, "Well, that is my quirky family, isn't it?" It can become a playful source of connection. Other times, it may simply be an act of acceptance and compassion.

# The Liminal Phase: Feeling the Grief

We have come to the place where the liminal moment of change is close at hand. Intellectual insight is always helpful in this process, but what seals the deal is the emotional transformation. A person may let himself feel the emotion that surrounds the specific shadow or real parent issue, and at some point may feel as though his heart is breaking. In some cases, he is experiencing this grief from the perspective (both emotionally and mentally) of a little boy. In the liminal work, this is very possible. In fact, it is this controlled regression back to a childlike experience that makes it possible to revisit these old wounds in a way that allows for healing. So, be patient with your strong man in these moments. He trusts you with a precious gift, that of revealing his tender vulnerability. There will be pockets of sorrow that need to be tapped and drained away. For many men this causes a deep ache that brings tears to his eyes. He may find himself weeping deeply over how disappointing shadow parent issues felt. He may find himself feeling more vulnerable and emotionally thin than normal and wonder, "What have I gotten myself into? I am falling apart." While it may seem counterintuitive, he actually gets better by temporarily feeling worse. The grief work is a process. It is not meant to be resolved in one or even several sessions. He may even do this type of work in conjunction with a trained therapist.

If he can stay with this process long enough, a strange thing will begin to occur. Feeling the pain that he has learned to deaden himself to for years provides an unexpected gift—he may feel alive in the midst of it. He feels alive because it is good to feel things (rather than stuffing his emotions), even those feelings that are uncomfortable and intense. Feelings that resonate in an authentic way have a life to them, even when painful.

In addition, in this process he becomes attuned to those aspects that he has kept shut off or at a distance for a long time. As a child, many of these intense feelings were beyond his ability to bear or understand. But now, as he welcomes that transformed part of himself back, there is an opportunity to reconnect and be revitalized. He must keep in mind that the grief is built on the foundation of life-affirming energy. Each time he delves deep enough, he ends up touching and engaging life-giving power. There may be a bitter sweetness to these feelings, though it is not self-pity. He learns to be gentle with himself and to validate the importance of feeling grief. There may be a sense of pride that he was able to face the pain he once thought was unbearable.

My own father could be a scary man at times. He could be surly, say hurtful things, and sometimes be physically overbearing. I have a poignant recollection that drives home how my shadow father felt for me. My nightly prayers would include things like, "Please keep the dogs safe, watch over the ten people in my family, make the world a nicer place," and, if it was a particularly bad day with my dad, I'd pray that one day I would be big enough to beat him up. I can look back now with adult eyes and see how frustrated, depressed, and alone my dad often felt. These feelings often came flying out of him, disguised as unexpected fits of anger. After working on our relationship for a number of years, I began to have more compassion for that part of him. There were measurable steps along the way to a better relationship.

Once, in my late twenties, I came back to town for a quick visit. My father and I were standing in the lobby of a hotel, and he said something that was dangerously close to the spirit of my worst shadow father recollection. In that moment, I felt my blood boil, memories of his antics from the past flooding my mind like scenes from a movie. I felt angry, really angry . . . and strangely, I recollected my prayer as a little boy.

Then I looked at my father—really looked at him. I saw a familiar expression on his face; it was so recognizable it took me off guard. My father looked scared; he was frightened of my grimace. Just then, I could see on my real father's face the same look that I had borne as a boy. I could remember how it was to be a scared kid in the presence of an angry other. The contorted image of my shadow father faded in that moment, as he seemed to age before my eyes, looking old and frail.

Being an intimidating force to my father did not make me feel powerful or triumphant, just nauseous. I felt myself soften and put my arm around his shoulder as we walked out of the hotel lobby. This moment was one for revelry, not for the near completion of a child's fantasy; it was the long over-due resetting of a perception. As we walked, my father asked if I had grown since my last visit. "No, Dad," I said, "I am nearly thirty; I stopped growing a long time ago." "Funny," he said, "you seem taller."

## ▶ Toolbox Tip: Anger as a Barrier for Grief

One of the most difficult things to do in the grief process is to stay with whatever comes up. One of the chief distractions is letting anger block the underlying sadness. The Ten Commandments of Growing Up Male state that all tender and vulnerable man emotions get funneled into sex or aggression, so it makes sense that these same coping skills are utilized here as well. One of the rules of thumb I tell clients is that while anger may alert you to the work that needs to be done, it is not always the underlying emotion that ultimately needs to be dealt with when it comes to grief. Instead, it is often about squeezing the sack of sadness and hurt until it is empty.

# Assimilation (Phase 3)

The last phase involves reentering the world with a new sense of inner peace regarding both shadow and real parents. The inner world has seen a significant transformation, but the work is not yet complete; in many ways, it is just the beginning of a new life. In any rite of transformation, the assim-ilation phase marks the start of a new identity, but this should not be con-fused with having mastered or fully realized all its subtle nuances. There are still important tasks left to do.

The last phase involves more transformation of the inner and outer worlds with two essential goals: (1) to further solidify the recently changed shadow image(s) of parents, and (2) to seek new types of relationships that do not involve real parents or shadow parent stand-ins but allow them to meet important needs from the past. While most people have encountered both shadow and real parents in the liminal phase, it is this continued work that allows these images to stay in their proper place. This entails keeping real parents from morphing back into shadow ones as a new type of relationship progresses. This is put to the test both with the real parents in the outside world and stand-ins who take their place. Second, by developing new relationships that feed the heart and mind, the prerequisite level of emotional sustenance can be met, making it possible to engage work and love in more healthy ways. The burden is taken off of the caregiver to make up for all that was not received in the formative years. Even as an adult, a person can seek out healthy ways to compensate for what was never received. In these last sections, I will highlight specific work that is associated with each of these tasks in the assimilation phase.

## The Assimilation Phase: What Actually Happens to the Shadow Parent(s)?

Some people will inevitably wonder what really happens to the shadow parent(s) carried inside: "Are they plucked from the psyche like a bad tooth, never to be a source of trouble again?" Shadow parents really don't disappear; they are a permanent part of our psychological makeup. In the best situations, they transform into more realistic versions of actual parents. The emphasis should be on what we choose to access: the shadow versions, which cause childlike regressions, or the real ones, which can guide interactions in work and love with more wisdom and compassion.

For some, the status of internal parents moves back and forth like a teeter-totter, never quite achieving solid ground. A common scenario is to make real gains through grief and acceptance (in the liminal phase), only to feel old, uncomfortable emotions arising yet again when in the presence of the actual parent(s) or stand-in(s). Under duress, or especially in the early stages of assimilation, there is a normal tendency to allow the more realistic version of the parent to backslide into a more shadowy one.

People often take "field trips" back home to put the staying power of their new, hard-won identities to the test. They may feel a mix of pride that so much hard work has yielded a new perspective on old relationships, yet also some trepidation about not knowing exactly how much pressure these new perspectives can withstand when back in old, familiar settings. What may feel like a firm stance can turn to feet of clay upon the discovery that parents have not moved forward on the same issues.

These initial visits may not yield all that was hoped for; in fact, some may feel deeply disappointed that though parents have not changed, they also haven't stood more firmly behind their own psychological gains. While some may feel discouraged, this is not a sign of failure; rather, it is a normal part of the process of making peace. Sometimes more challenges need to be encountered for the old images to coalesce into a solid form. Additional emotional work, as highlighted in the liminal phase, may need to be done. One does not pass through transformation of the inner world in a linear way; the rite of transformation that governs the inner world is often circular, going through the differing phases as many times as needed to complete the journey. The assimilation phase allows additional skills to be mastered in order that changes may become permanent.

In the assimilation process, one begins to pick up certain abilities that make it easier to function in the real world when interacting with others. These include learning to turn down the volume on the intense emotional reactions that, left unchecked, can be the culprits that quickly turn compassion and understanding with difficult others into an emotional wrestling match. Often people walk away from encounters with parents or stand-ins when they lose their cool, wishing they had not taken the extra step that sent them over the edge.

There is a trial-and-error approach when monitoring the level of reactivity, being aware of hot-button topics that need to be handled with special care. In these encounters, there is a need to find a source of grounding, because in all honesty, there will be moments of strain. Being grounded means standing firmly in your best self, the self that is connected to the adult world of functioning. The decisions made at crucial turning points often dictate the outcomes of encounters. Not being grounded is like slid-ing back into a regressed form of relating; one becomes too emotional, not seeing things clearly, or with tunnel vision, placing parents back in their for-mer shadow form.

Emotional grounding can be thought of as the adult stance, the one that enables you to understand multiple perspectives and gives you access to compassion, wisdom, and, when need be, a measure of firmness. An emo-tionally grounded person is like a wise old grandfather or mother who knows how to avoid the pitfalls of old traps and is working in the best inter-est of everyone. In fact, one of the ways to stay grounded is by picturing in your mind's eye a person who represents those types of qualities. One may make the commitment to follow this standard in these interactions when confused or when intensity gets high: "What would my wise old grandfa-ther/mother do here?"

Another form of mental grounding can be used during these encounters, especially if one begins to falter and the shadow image of a parent begins to loom on the horizon. This skill involves grounding yourself by hanging on tightly to a parent's most endearing aspects: frailty, elderly status, sincerity, their love for you, your love for them, their imperfections, and so on. One does not let go of these aspects; they are simultaneously the lifeline and the shield that keeps you connected to the parent and fends off would-be emo-tional reactivity that threatens to sabotage the relationship.

There are always decision points in intense visits with parents that involve reenacting old dramas or taking the more difficult approach of play-ing out the new internal scripts. To do the latter requires your best self, even if the struggle initially feels palpable. After tense moments have passed, there will be the sensation of having made it over the hump, and coasting down the hill makes it feel worth the effort. Grounding can be reflected in your resolve for doing this important work: you want more than anything to have peace inside, and you and possibly your caregiver stretch in these dif-ficult moments. You stretch because you don't want to pass on the same old hurt to those you love, certainly not your own kids . . .

## ▶ Toolbox Tip: Preparing for Parental Visits

Some people find a preemptive emotional strategy useful as they prepare for an anticipated stressful encounter with a parent. This includes taking special care to relax and be in a good place emotionally before engaging parents. Doing reconciliation work is hard enough without adding other unnecessary stresses. Not taking steps toward good self-care may cause oversensitivity and overreaction, conjuring shadow parents back into existence.

Staying grounded and using proper "reparative skills" also helps during these visits. Reparative work is by definition owning responsibility for your part of a conflict and taking the proper steps to make amends. Sometimes this involves action in the midst of a discussion or argument, when an offense is detected by one's own self-monitoring or through seeing the reactions of the other person. Reparative work may also occur after the fact, when tempers have cooled and enough space allows for clearer reflection. In this case, reparation through phone calls, e-mails, or letters expresses the desire to make things right and take another try. A heartfelt "I am sorry" or "I wish I didn't say it that way" can go a long way.

Even though a man has gone through the steps of letting go of his shadow parents, reconciling the new, proper image in actual situations takes time. What may have felt like a challenging trial run when encountering the shadow parent in recollections stirs up another set of intense feelings when actually interacting in the real world. The hope is that each new encounter will encourage progress, allowing the real parent image to become more rooted and less likely to regress to its previous shadow form. This continued work has an impact on people; after all, they are no longer operating from an emotionally laden internal script. After many sessions, there is a time when the shadow image becomes more solid, and reactions are significantly decreased to manageable levels.

When perceptions of our real parents are firmly rooted in the inner realm, and they act as healthy guides for interactions in the outer world with others, a strange thing may occur. Some experience a sense of sadness when the shadow parent permanently fades away. This may seem odd given that so much hurt, sadness, and anger is tied to them—maybe there should be a series of celebrations instead. But as human beings, we can experience a complexity of feelings that involve a part of us feeling joy and relief that we're finally free, while another part of us is sad when we realize that so much of our lives has been bound and guided by shadow parents. They often inadvertently helped choose our clothes, romantic partners, careers, values, and opinions. Right or wrong, for some they have supplied the emotional fervor that underlies political and social causes.

Where would we be without the shadow parents? Better yet, *who* would we be without them? There is a sense of loss that goes with passing the reins of leadership from the shadow parents into our own hands. For many this comes with a mix of excitement and terror. It means we cannot blame them for old hurts and wounds anymore, or for future mistakes in work and love. We have reached an age of psychological accountability for our choices. This is the psychological place where a boy becomes a man and a girl becomes a woman. Many who reach this milestone know that the life they carve from here on is truly their own. There is a sense of ownership like never before—and that is worth getting excited about!

## ▶ Toolbox Tip: Healing as a Process

For some, the course of healing outlined in this chapter may feel like it starts making a difference immediately; for others, the cycle will need to be revisited from time to time, and it might take years to find a deeper peace. However, we should not think about this in terms of crossing the proverbial finish line: "No more pain from the past ever again." Instead, it is a process that is engaged when needed, always steadily moving forward.

Sometimes this means going back and forth between the three phases of separation, liminal, and assimilation when more work is called for. A person could be tempted to believe "All the work is done now," only to discover that he is being invited to a deeper level of healing by new issues that arise in the areas of work and love. For some, this will be a source of frustration: "Haven't I dealt with this stuff before? Will I ever be done with this process?!!!" People discover that sometimes the huge chunks of the past that keep us bound to unhappiness are chipped away one section at a time. And even when these boulders are removed, we will occasionally stumble across pebbles from the past. We are sometimes invited to revisit our work in this area for more fine-tuning.

## The Assimilation Phase: Seeking Relationships That Will Fill the Void

Moving the shadow parent to a more stable state is one goal in the assimilation phase, but there is another: seeking out new types of relationships to help fill the void of what was not received in the formative years. Part of reentering the world includes reorienting a person's internal compass toward those who can supply some of his emotional needs, instead of continuing the endless personalization-pursuit cycle that leaves one empty-handed and empty-hearted. When a man gets to that place, no longer expecting shadow or real parents to be responsible for his emotional needs, half the battle is won. The new mantra is "I will seek new relationships that nurture those parts of me that need it." This may occur in the context of his relationship with you, but also with a therapist, friend, or peer. We need to realize that more than one person can fulfill this role. It would be too taxing to demand that one individual fill all of these needs.

It is also important to note that in these new relationships, he can fulfill some of the needs he missed out on in the past, but not all of them. Some aspects from growing up have to be accepted as losses and released. For instance, we walk the delicate balance of having some needs met that reactivate those frozen parts of us; this allows us to continue on our way toward mature relations with others and ourselves, which is the main goal of this phase.

However, certain aspects cannot be recaptured and should not be sought in our relationships now. If we are not careful, we can create a situation of desperate false hope in which we strive to get all those previously denied childlike fantasies met in our adult relationships now. In fact, we can set up cycles in our relationships that place us back in those old familiar and often disappointing scenarios. For some who begin to feel the healing and corrective experience of having someone meet their needs like never before, it is understandable that a part of them wonders exactly how far this can go. Sometimes childhood fantasies get transferred from parents to their new, more fulfilling relationships.

A man spoke of his very difficult relationship with his father. Growing up, his attempts at affection and connection were often rebuffed in painful ways. Over many months of therapy, he had come to accept that connection would never be the way he wished. In one of these painful moments of realization, he blurted out his wish that I could be his father. We discussed how there is a natural inclination to seek out available others when uncovering old wounds from the past. It even stirs up old hopes and dreams from childhood.

The hard part was that he could realistically expect me (or any other available person) to supply some of what he needed to get the emotional frozen part of him unstuck, but the fantasy of having me as a father was transferring old hopes and wishes from his old dad onto his new symbolic one. If he could not have his old father, then he would find a new one to replace him. What was missing was letting go of the deeper, childlike fantasy that someone would assume the role of caregiver.

If he were to hang on to this hope, it would prevent him from making the ultimate transition, that of becoming a father (caregiver) to himself. His task was to seek out and enjoy the good care of others but utilize that emotional nurturance to adjust his degree of expectations from others. He could in turn learn to care for himself in a new way that reflected giving up old hopes that would never happen and by doing so gain both a new level of emotional connection and independence.

Transitioning to the adult world is often hard enough to do, even in the best of circumstances. One of the things that our new nurturing relationships do is supply us with enough of what we need to make this transition. Loving care from others allows us to face the inevitabilities of life, and that includes the loss of things that will never be. Arrested development does not let a person see that certain expectations, hopes, and wishes should not be met. Good care is a tool that helps set us free from childlike hopes and wishes, not something that gives us license to stay stuck. While we may not be able to fulfill childlike fantasies, have all our needs gratified on demand, or even, as in the case above, have new parents replace the old ones, we can feel the healing impact of caring people who help us make the transition to a new level of maturity. It may feel as though ointment is being placed on old wounds from the past, and depending on the depth of hurt, it may take some time to heal. It takes practice to learn how much we can realistically expect of others, whether friends, romantic partners, or therapists.

## ▶ Toolbox Tip: Landscape of the Inner World

We carry many people around with us in our psyches and hearts. Some, as we have seen, are the shadow parents. In the best situations, these are transformed into more real versions of caregivers. They are a permanent part of who we are, but it is important to note that shadow parents are not the only people who reside within.

Most of us need at least one good person in our lives to help us survive the psychological bumps that go with growing up. This can be a family member, a best friend, or a teacher—anyone who touched your life in a special way. These people occupy space in our psyches as well. As we grow into adulthood and beyond, the hope is that we collect more of these people in our psyches, ones who are a healthy source of support and who will stand with us in tough times. It is like we have access to an internal village of people we can turn to when needed—we just have to remember they are there.

One of my patients once discussed an upcoming operation about which he was very anxious. He was more fearful of the aftermath than the actual procedure. He had the recollection of being a small boy in the hospital undergoing a series of procedures over a number of months. While he had visitors, this was a period in his life when he felt most alone. Even though he was much older now, he feared that he would experience the same sense of painful seclusion. We talked about the many people who had touched his life and how they had become a permanent part of him—people he had access to, even in his hospital bed. In moments of duress it is tempting to feel set adrift, alone in the vast ocean of life, while in reality, we have a life-line to the good people we carry inside even when they are a thousand miles way.

## Care for Self and Others: The Emergence of a New Voice from Within

As a result of reshaping shadow parents and receiving good, steady care from others, a man begins to feel the emergence of newly defined skills— the ability to better care for himself and for others. I am not just talking about the ability to do his own laundry and pick up around the house; it's more like the ability to be a caregiver for himself, providing his own self-directed sense of support and challenge to succeed in work and be there for those he loves.

This can take the form of being a better romantic partner, parent, family member, and friend. In business, a man draws from his inner resources to make connections and negotiate deals successfully. Shadow images that were once stumbling blocks for relationships and achievement have found more peace, and when they make their presence known again, there is a keener awareness of how to deal with them in a swifter way.

When life's inevitable difficulties need to be faced, his new inner voice emerges, one based on the culmination of good care received by others. The good people he has experienced in his life have taken root in his inner world. These people—men, women, romantic partners, friends, and family— encourage him to move forward. These voices replace the accusatory shadow parents who have held sway for so long. Peace with the shadow parents is ultimately about changing a person's inner landscape; what once was shadowy and filled with pockets of pain now emerges as a different environment. The inner realm becomes a rich resource, a personal sanctuary, not a barrier for his interactions in work and love as before; he carries the new images of those who balance out the past and help negotiate the present.

While never outgrowing the deeper need or desire for connection, a man who has felt the presence of those people in his life can now fulfill in a more genuine way some of his cherished notions of being a man—those involving strength and independence. However, this emerges not as bravado or emotional distance, but rather as the ability to live comfortably in his own skin as he recognizes the ebb and flow of all his important relationships.

Sometimes this is about being very connected with those he loves. A man can be more fully present, even in painful emotional situations, because the clutter of his own past has been sorted. Till then, hearing others' tender stories too closely reminds him of his own and acts as an inconvenient distraction in moments when his full attention is needed. Instead, a newfound strength enables him to use the recollection of his own pain as a way to understand the hurt of others, thereby deepening the bond of connection.

He knows the power of being seen and heard because he has experienced them both firsthand, and he can extend those same nurturing qualities to others. Other times, a man who has transformed his inner world can enjoy the rich moments of solitude, feeling connected to all of his parts without the former inner barricades to bridle the flow. Before the shadow work, being alone may have smacked of aloofness, melancholy, or disconnection.

So much of the internal scenery of this new life comes through making peace with the past and then injecting fresh elements that are good for the psyche and heart. From this process of reconciling the past and resetting the course of the future, a new type of relationship with self and others emerges. These experiences become the foundation upon which he not only becomes his own man but makes choices to do so in healthy ways.

# Conclusion

In this chapter we looked at healing the relationships with the shadow parents and the real parents. This can be a long-term process that for some may not only occupy much time and effort but may need to be revisited throughout one's life. The goal is to transform the painful parts of the inner world and then add friends, family, and romantic partners who provide different types of experiences.

Bad feelings toward shadow parents are a part of what is left behind in the primal space of transformation. The shadow parent(s) have begun to take on a three-dimensional appearance now, no longer monsters wreaking havoc. Instead, they are seen as real people now, taking on identities beyond that of personal caregivers; there is the realization that they are and have always been individuals with their own hopes, wishes, disappointments, and limitations. This understanding helps people to break the damaging personalization-pursuit equation when they begin to consider that it is really not all about them. Not having what you needed as a child was not a marker of a lack of worth or being unlovable. Now that healing has begun, we can add the words "forgiveness" and "compassion" to our new vocabulary when considering caregivers and ourselves.

Many who do shadow parent work feel they can shake off the proverbial family curse of failed relationships, unhappy offspring, or always getting passed over for promotions. I think the most central experience is a greater sense of ownership of their lives. In Chapter 11, we will look at how the right "guardian" is a pivotal and essential connection, both for its power to help heal past psychological wounds and lend assistance in helping boys and men become their *own* man.

# CHAPTER CUES

1. Rites of transformation can be applied to the inner world of shadow parents.

2. The three phases of inner transformation include separation, liminal, and assimilation.

3. The goal of shadow parent work is to rewrite the inner landscape of the heart and psyche. This includes transforming the shadow version of a parent into a more realistic one based on a compassionate understanding of him or her as an individual beyond the role as caregiver.

4. The inner landscape is also changed by adding the presence of new people and their good care. This often heals the wounds that the shadow parents and subsequent stand-ins could not.

5. A central part of making peace with the past and moving forward is learning about what can be expected in new nurturing relationships; that is, a key guideline for caring relationships is that they should point the person toward more mature functioning, not reinforce childlike hopes and fantasies.

6. When the inner world is changed, the outer world will also be affected. A new, healthier script for the relationship with the self and others is formed and subsequently acts as a guide.

# PART IV

# WHAT EVERY MAN NEEDS FROM A WOMAN, BUT IS AFRAID TO ASK

# 9

# The V Spot:
# Castrating the Man You Love

I realize that "Castrating the Man You Love" may seem like an odd title for a chapter in a book geared toward understanding men. Most people want to do just the opposite; they want to be the emotional and physical Viagra that propels their men to new heights. Or, if you are a family member or friend, you want to provide emotional support that deepens the connection between you in significant ways.

When we talk about castrating your man, we don't actually mean removing his genitals. Instead, the topics covered in this chapter refer to unintended slights that strike at the very core of a man's sense of vulnerability—his V Spot, if you will. The result of "stepping on" his V Spot is symbolic castration because it may leave a man feeling diminished or separated from his inherent power as a male. He may feel belittled or misunderstood in an extreme way; or, when being compared to others, he may feel that he doesn't measure up in your eyes.

Remember that *Seinfeld* episode when George is off on a weekend getaway with a would-be love interest? He finishes a swim in cold water and is changing clothes when, much to his horror, the woman comes in and sees him naked for the first time. She looks at him and is just surprised . . . at first. Then she looks down to his nether region, smirks with an unforgiving look, and leaves the room. George, realizing that the cold water has wreaked havoc on him, reducing his manhood, yells out in his own defense, "It's the shrinkage! It's the shrinkage!" The rest of the weekend she gives George the cold shoulder.

A man who has his V Spot exploited can feel a lot like George—it can be a "teenie weenie" moment. He feels misunderstood, small, and insignificant. He wants to say, "Hey, that's not all there is to me. I am just temporarily incapacitated due to the 'shrinkage' of the circumstances." However, it is difficult to recapture what feels lost. In his mind, there will always be that image of someone smirking at his shrinkage. He fears that he will never be looked at the same way, having lost the respect of someone who is important to him. Most romantic partners would indignantly say, "I would never want that to happen, much less make him feel small on purpose!" The unfortunate thing is that when a V Spot event occurs, even when the comment is not said in a spirit of meanness, there can be troubling effects just the same. In this chapter we will look at an important aspect of the secret lives of men: their V Spots and the "teenie weenie moments" that cause them pain.

# V Spots

V Spots are places of extreme vulnerability for men. The exact locale of a V spot is based on an individual's own unique history and what has caused him the most pain with regards to being a man. Given what we have looked at so far—the Ten Commandments of Growing Up Male, the Peter Pan Man, Lost Boys, and shadow parents—it's understandable why men pick up some painful baggage along the way.

However, the V Spot is unique because of all the aspects involved in being a man, this is his most sensitive. To damage it is like hitting the rawest of nerves. Sometimes men express this type of pain through rage that masks a deeper hurt. They may turn blue in the face yelling, but that outward intensity is a reflection of the inner emotional storm. Other times when a

V Spot is struck, a man will feel like his legs turn to jelly. He goes *plop* right to the ground, like someone knocked him out.

The mere existence of men's V Spots does not mean they are fragile, insecure beings or babies, it just means they are human. This is an important aspect of the secret lives of men: as much as they would like to think that the laws of emotional gravity don't apply to them, everyone carries tender places inside that can bring them down—even the strongest of people. (I should mention in passing that women have their own versions of V Spots as well. That is, they feel separated from their own power when a vulnerable area is struck. They have their own histories and hurts related to being a woman that are also sensitive.)

The V Spot is usually constructed over time through repeated, intense experiences that are emotionally damaging. In extreme cases, this can involve maltreatment, abuse, or neglect. Some in the area of men's psychology suggest that even the *normal* ways boys are raised are actually chockfull of opportunities to build V Spots. Each damaging encounter is like shoving pain, frustration, and disappointment into a sack that a man carries on his shoulders, and wrapped around the opening of this pack and keeping its contents out of sight from the view of the world is a leather strap known as *shame*. Shame adds significantly to the creation of a V Spot.

Shame is different from guilt, though the two are often confused. Guilt involves being remorseful for something you have done. It is healthy and corrective because it guides a person toward more appropriate behavior. For instance, if you hurt someone you love, the natural and healthy thing to do is to feel bad about it. It is the moral and psychological compass that says, "Make amends to the person and do better next time." Shame, on the other hand, does not focus on bad behavior; instead, it centers on the very core sense of an individual's personal worth and value. The bad behavior in question is only a mere reflection of a deeper, much more troubling malady. Shaming messages carry a poignant memo stating that you are worthless and beyond the hope of ever receiving love from anyone. As you might imagine, shame is a very heavy emotional burden.

Besides being unhealthy, shame is counterproductive with regards to changing someone. Even if you make the most shaming comments you can imagine to a man, believing it will change who he is, you will eventually discover the only thing that is really different is his awareness about what not to share with the world. Shame does nothing to change his inner self for the better. In fact, the usual response to a shame assault is to psychologically shut down concerning that particular area, because to dwell upon those things only makes a person uncomfortable. This approach to dealing with shame does not promote the introspection needed to sift through an experience in a way that leads to a behavior change. Instead of working through the situation, emotions are left in a raw and intense state. All those troubling thoughts and feelings just sit there, and the man in question makes a mental note never to explore that area of his mind and heart again: "Note to self: never share vulnerable feelings with anyone ever again. Note to self: better destroy that last message about what not to share, just to be on the safe side."

"Keep Out" and "Abandoned Property" signs are posted in that quadrant of his psyche, in the hopes this will permanently protect the shamed area. However, it is certain that, sooner or later, someone will stumble across the forbidden zone by chance. Maybe after ten, twenty, or thirty years, this once-abandoned territory will be trod upon by a stranger who doesn't know that a shame-filled massacre occurred here, and the area in question is off-limits.

You never know when you might come across one of these areas. You could be driving along with your new romantic interest on a sunny Sunday afternoon, birds singing and music playing. In the course of a conversation that is meant to deepen all the other good stuff going on, you unexpectedly witness a rush of intense feelings from your man. "Wow," you think, "he really overreacted to what I said; he is very touchy and sensitive. Poor thing, he must be insecure." To those who have not received the proper V Spot recognition training, these conclusions are the only ones that make sense.

Yet, for all its trouble, shame plays an important part in man training. It is perceived as the ultimate tool to make a boy or a man fly right. Once, at a university meeting, I heard a colleague say that so-and-so was not performing to his full capacity as a student. The solution, he suggested, was to "Get in his face and shame him for not being a man." I agree that being a straight shooter with people is a healthy and important way to help them reach their full potential. I have had my share of direct discussions (also known as "Come to Jesus" talks throughout the southern part of the United States) with students to help get them back on track.

However, the difference here is that calling someone's worth as a human being into question hits at the very core of who he is. Men especially have intense emotional reactions to being shamed. It is not because they are wired differently; it has more to do with a legacy of man-training that relies heavily on the use of it. This is why the V Spot is such a potentially emotionally loaded area.

Another reason shame is so potent is because there is a central message in man-training that males are not supposed to let things affect them, send them over the edge, or emotionally stop them. Even harsh treatment or tragic consequences should be met with the stoic resolve of taking it on the chin. If you look at some of the great works of art in Western culture, often the central male character portrays this heroic stoicism even in the face of chaos and death.

A more recent example of this involves Frederic Remington's work; he was one of the nineteenth- and early twentieth-century artists who brought the Wild West to life in paintings and sculpture. In most of his intense scenes, the hero is portrayed as calm and collected, even though all hell is breaking loose around him. One painting portrays a daring escape from Indians, another, a shootout with foes. One of the interesting things in Remington's style is that you have to look at the animals in the paintings to get a real read of the intensity of the moment. Many times the animals look fear-struck and overwhelmed, but not the cowboys—they are emotional rocks. One of my favorite Remington paintings is entitled *Aiding a Comrade* (originally, *Beyond First Aid*). In this painting, three cowboys ride side by side while pursued dangerously close by Indians. One of the comrades is struck and, falling from his horse, about to hit the ground and meet certain death. There is an eerie look of tranquility on the faces of the two who still remain in the saddle and also on that of the one about to perish.

A way of summing up how shame relates to V Spots is that an initial combination of shame and pain creates a V Spot. There is then lingering potential for feeling even more shame when the man allows this emotionally wounded part to affect him. This is a tough situation many men feel uncomfortable about acknowledging to themselves, much less discussing with someone else. Unprocessed shame casts a cloud of confusion upon situations (see Relationship Red Zone below) that can cause men to feel paranoid and unsure about who to trust.

From the sometimes-suspicious male perspective of struggling for power over themselves and others, the V Spot can be a potential doorway to a feared exploitation. If revealed to the wrong person, he believes it will be used against him. Consequently, there won't be a lot of men wearing T-shirts that say, "Ask me about my V Spot." Instead, men will react to V Spots by keeping them from view. This restriction may even apply to his closest friends, family, and romantic partner.

It is a big leap to reveal this aspect of the secret shoe box. It is very well guarded. Most of the time, V Spots are discussed only after the fact, when the direness of a situation demands an explanation. A friend or romantic partner may be on the verge of packing the relationship in when he makes the decision to open up and discuss the legacy of why he reacted with such intensity. The real story of disappointments and old wounds that still fester may then emerge.

## RELATIONSHIP RED ZONE:
### V Spot Fog

Most people have heard the phrase "emotionally arrested." It may sound like something straight out of a psychology textbook; well, that's probably because it is. But what does it mean exactly? Sometimes people experience events that are very emotionally damaging and traumatic. When these events occur and are not sorted through, a part of the person can get emotionally stuck at the moment the event occurred; they get arrested in all the pain and emotional confusion, like some sort of fog has descended upon them. They don't see with any clarity what is around them; they feel disoriented, powerless, and small.

After a moment or two of grappling in absolute darkness, the normal response is to try to run away through that fog as quickly as possible. After all, it is scary in there! But, as in the case of the creation of the V Spot, prematurely running from the situation gives people a false sense that they have safely escaped its clutches. Sometimes people feel they have purchased a foolproof insurance plan against the traumatic event or topic by keeping it locked away from the view of themselves and others. They think, "As long as I never talk about it or even think about it, I will never experience that again." But in the case of a V Spot, we have a tendency to stumble back upon our old hurts and emotional wounds. When that occurs, it is like picking up right where you left off. Some people even begin to experience the same emotional and physical sensations that occurred during the event, like a flashback.

I bring this up because men who have had traumatic V Spot events can experience this type of situation when they are suddenly taken off guard by returning to the emotionally arrested areas in their hearts and minds. They may feel like they are in a

V Spot fog to varying degrees. The telltale sign of this occurring is when a grown man suddenly appears much younger than he actually is. His facial expressions may look like a young boy's, and his reactions may not be those of an adult. Instead, he may seem childlike in his level of defensiveness, caution, tone of voice, and actions.

The first time you witness a V Spot fog, you may be thinking to yourself, "This does not seem like my man at all; he is acting very strange." Being the other party witnessing someone in the V Spot fog can be difficult and confusing. When reflecting on the situation later, you may be able to identify the exact point when the fog began to set in. To help neutralize this situation for him, you will utilize attunement skills we have already discussed, like staying sturdy in the midst of witnessing someone else's pain, protecting their vulnerability, and so on.

For now, just focus on some of the ways the man you care about shows he is in a V Spot fog. For some, the specifics will automatically come to mind. Others may have to work at it a bit by considering the types of thoughts he seems to have (that you are out to hurt him), the defensive maneuvers he employs (telling you he doesn't want to talk about it and then shutting down or escaping by himself), or the emotions he expresses (anger, edginess, sadness). The upside of doing this type of exercise is that you will be better prepared the next time the fog rolls in.

# Empathic Failures

Before we discuss some specific examples of V Spot encounters, let us look at a related topic that makes V Spot fouls so powerfully destructive. Recall from an earlier chapter the concept of attunement. Remember how attunement manifests in various ways, such as the "repackager" for difficult situations. A repackager's job is to make a difficult situation easier for another through understanding and explaining difficult circumstances. In moments of personal crisis, being attuned to another person and what they need is very important. Sometimes this may involve things like offering a comforting word, while other times it may be listening without interruption. These types of attuned responses help a person in a bad emotional place put the pieces back together, and usually the result is that the crisis abates and the person feels soothed and restored.

The opposite of attunement is empathically failing someone. Empathic failure entails being out-of-sync with another's thoughts and feelings when it is vital that you understand their inner world and respond accordingly. These opportunities can occur when someone is under adverse circumstances, like lots of stress, or when they want to share an important new personal accomplishment or significant interpersonal happening. Empathic failures can arise when someone needs you to understand their pain or joy and you are unable to do so.

As powerful as attunement is as an agent of help, one can take that same force and bend it in the other direction through empathic failures. Just as attunement can add to a person psychologically or emotionally, empathic failures potentially subtract. Being out of sync can make a bad situation worse. The upset person can feel even more banged up when they reach out for assistance and someone drops the ball.

Empathic failures can also happen if you do not respond empathically when someone has important news to share with you; this can sour the special moment. This might involve getting married, a new job, or finding the perfect pair of pumps. The one who fails might be sidetracked by well-meaning concern or be too focused on some detail and comment: "Please tell me you're not going to marry that loser!" "The new job will be a long commute" or "Those shoes make your feet look too big!" The failed person often feels like saying, "Can't you just be happy for me?"

One can be out of sync in various degrees, sometimes a little and sometimes a lot. We probably all know how the differing degrees of empathic failures feel. If someone is just slightly off, people may say, "Well, that is not what I need from you right now; do this instead." In these cases, an attentive listener may make the needed microadjustments and sail on from there. However, when the margin between what was needed and what was received is too great (this varies by person and situation), it can lead to a real sense of being hurt and let down by someone who is counted on. The rule of thumb to keep in mind is, the bigger the miss, the more painful and derailing the empathic failure is. When important relationships (like with parents or partners) are characterized by frequent empathic failures, especially in key moments of vulnerability, it can lead to psychological damage.

I worked with a client who had repeated dreams of running out of gas in his car. Sometimes this would occur during normal functioning, like pulling out of the driveway, while other times he would run out of fuel in more dire situations, such as when he had to accelerate to get onto the freeway. This man was dreaming in symbolic terms. He had a history marred by caregivers who failed him in some painful ways when he needed them most. His response in life was to always be on the verge of personally running out of gas. This could be seen in his job history, his romantic relationships, and even in therapy. When push came to shove, he did not have the emotional resources to feel confident in stepping on the accelerator to move ahead. In contrast to his history of repeated empathic failures, what he needed when growing up was someone to fill up the tank during the tough times. He needed someone to extend empathy and understanding.

Adding to the complexity of understanding empathic failures is that there are a number of different ways of being out of sync with what a person needs. For instance, a person may empathically fail someone by focusing on solutions to a problem instead of just listening to the person's pain or confusion. The offended party may feel like saying, "Oh, please, just shut up and listen to me; I don't need you to solve the problem; I just want to vent to someone." Sometimes empathic failures occur when caregivers or romantic partners are too busy to notice someone is in a bad way. Instead, they may brush it off as unimportant or casual talk, not pursuing or paying close enough attention to the situation.

Another version of empathic failures involves a well-meaning person missing the subtle nuances of what is being conveyed because they think about the problem from their own frame of reference. They may think, "Well, this is how I would feel if it were me." People forget in those moments to try to think from the other person's point of view instead of their own. To be empathically in tune means to understand the other person's world; people commit an empathic failure when they impose their own experiences upon someone else's feelings or experiences.

The intensity of a situation may also cause an empathic failure to occur. Sometimes well-meaning people are uncomfortable in moments of crisis. When others open up in a way that reveals their pain, it can catch a person off guard. Hearing someone's raw emotion can be difficult enough when you get a heads-up about it coming, but sometimes a V Spot is suddenly revealed. It appears like a flash of lightning with full-force intensity. When this occurs, people may wish to gloss over the situation as quickly as possible. A likely response is something like, "Everything will be okay," which is received by the person in distress as, "Please shut up; you are making me uncomfortable!"

Also, the anticipation of too much discomfort at seeing another's pain can lead to empathic failures. The person may imagine how a conversation may go and potentially feel afraid that they cannot handle the situation or may not be strong enough to manage their own uneasiness and still attend to the other person. These people hope in their hearts this is just a phase the child (or adult) is going through, and that it will soon disappear. Sometimes these fears stem from a person's experiences of empathic failures in their own childhoods. They may not know how to handle these emotion-filled situations because no one was able to give them proper care. (Better ways to handle these types of situations are given in the next two chapters on providing positive feedback and being a guardian for your man.)

Jack recalled that when he was a boy, his mother could not manage crises very well. If Jack was upset, he would hear his mother say, in a panicked way, "It will be okay . . . it will be okay . . . you'll see." And that ended the conversation. She would then nervously clear the dinner table or begin straightening things in the room. Jack learned over time that his mother could not be counted on for any real emotional support in moments of personal crisis.

He often initially reacted by feeling guilty for making his mother seem anxious about his problems; however, later, when he had time to think, he also felt unsupported and angry toward her. Jack thought her inability to be there for him was a reflection of her lack of concern. When Jack became an adult, he realized that his mother had been shortchanged by her mother and grandmother in a similar way while she was growing up, and this helped him to not take her behavior personally.

Unfortunately, in very harsh situations, the level of empathic failure is taken to an even more damaging level. This is usually based on assumptions about how men are always supposed to be stoic, unaffected by even the most troubling personal circumstances. Some caregivers see the child's (or adult's) vulnerability in moments of crisis and are repulsed by it. They see it as weakness, something boys and men are not supposed to have. In these cases, an individual might resort to the rationalization that they must prepare their boy or man to survive in the "real world," and allowing him to be "weak" only does him a disservice. In worst-case scenarios, the male feels shamed or humiliated for being vulnerable. He also quickly learns to cover up vulnerabilities and not show them to others. Parents and partners are lulled into the false belief that the "weakness" has been purged by using what they think is a tough-love approach. Yet nothing could be further from the truth. Remember, shame assaults and empathic failures don't toughen people up; instead, those experiences weaken them.

## Empathic Failures Part II: Not Seeing the Man You Love

While many types of empathic failures involve being out of sync with a person's needs in moments of crisis, there is another version that involves failing to honor the authentic qualities that make a man his own unique person. These types of empathic failures can be thought of as not truly valuing the man you love for who he is. We all have a psychological need to be genuinely appreciated for just being ourselves—no fronts or personas. Lasting relationships are based on the type of care where a person can share the whole package of who he is—the good, the bad, and the ugly—and still have that important person always there to say she loves him.

Sometimes the worst empathic failures occur when the genuine building blocks of a man's identity are either ignored or devalued. That is, the core aspects of who he is as a man go unappreciated or even worse when revealed to another. Often this can happen accidentally, when a partner or parent fails to recognize or acknowledge a genuine aspect of who a man is. But sometimes in relationships, this type of empathic failure can also be the fodder for really bad fights, as in the heat of anger, you may feel compelled to go for the jugular, knowing exactly what to say or do to deeply wound him. Needless to say, those types of attacks are relationship killers. Let's look at some specific ways at how not valuing who he really is can be wounding. We will start with a parent's expectations for a boy, but the spirit of these interactions can also easily parallel a wife, partner, or friend's hopes for a man.

It is normal for parents expecting a child to begin to imagine how their child will be. It is perfectly normal for parents to begin to daydream about how the child may grow up and add significance to their own lives. They may imagine the smell of their baby and the opportunity to cuddle him (or her) and how that will enhance the parents' sense of being alive. They may think about family trips and special moments that will be shared. Parents may even wonder about all the things they will learn from being a parent and connecting with their child. When they find out the gender of the child, it adds another dimension to these fantasies. All this is normal.

But this type of imagining can become damaging when the parents begin to focus too much on how their child will make up for their own emotional wounds and deficits. They may imagine that "this child will love me and be a source of support for me," unlike their own parents were or significant other is now. They may envision specific scenarios in which the child's main purpose is to meet their own emotional needs. They finally have someone who is their unquestioning ally, always agreeing with them; or they may believe they have found a companion who will make them feel special or take the loneliness and hurt away.

When these types of situations arise, it can easily impair a would-be-caregiver's ability to validate his/her son as his own man. When there is a break with what was anticipated in the imaginary world, the parent may think, "Hey! You're not supposed to be that way! I am mad at you! You were brought into this world to meet my needs." In these situations, the boy experiences an intense empathic failure. What he needed was someone to value the genuine parts of his budding notion of being a man. Instead, he feels devalued for being who he really is. Consequently, he feels torn inside; a part of him feels compelled to hide the true parts of himself that displease his parents, while another part of him wants to become his own man. These situations become even worse when a caregiver (male or female) has significant issues related to men and masculinity that go unresolved and unchecked. In these situations, the child will be at risk for receiving the brunt of this damage.

Let's consider some examples of parents whose own unresolved issues have a very negative effect on their sons. They entangle their boys in their own personal troubles. A father who feels significant insecurities related to being a man will sometimes demand that his son make up for these failings through "appropriate" actions and behavior. This may include demanding that the boy strive for achievements the father could not accomplish himself, couching this in terms of the boy not being a real man until he succeeds: "When you are a star athlete, get an education, or make lots of money, then I can give my blessing that you are a good man."

In this very damaging situation, the father unconsciously does not want the boy to ever measure up, because if he does, the father would have no other way to disguise his own shortcomings. The father sees himself in his son's weakness, and he confronts aspects of his son's personality that he has not resolved in himself. If the father cannot purge those gnawing feelings inside of himself, he will do it externally through controlling his son. In the father's view, he is trying to toughen up the boy or make him a success.

Female caregivers can also harm a boy through extreme empathic failures related to not valuing him for his own person. Mothers can influence the way their sons see men in general. A mother who tells her son that all men cannot be trusted, or that they are hypersexual, or that they will leave when you need them most may pass on these skewed messages to her child. One day the boy realizes, "Hey, I am a member of that corrupt gender as well; I must be doomed to live out my mother's prophecies."

Such a boy experiences an empathic failure because his own mother casts doubt on his worth as a man. Mothers can also have fantasies that they will raise their sons to be the kind of emotionally responsive male caregiver or romantic partner whom they themselves wished for but never found. In this case, the son is asked to cater to the wishes of his mother, who has not worked through her conflicts concerning men. The boy becomes her "emotional partner." This ultimately blocks the boy from investing this type of emotional energy in age-appropriate peers or romantic interests. Sometimes mothers intensify the damage done to their sons by making guilt-inducing remarks or "threats" about looking elsewhere for support or lulling him into thinking that being her emotional partner is a special honor.

The effects of these troubling occurrences can follow a man into his adult relationships with women. If a woman is in the habit of making guilt-inducing accusations about him not doing enough for those he loves, he can easily cave to her demands. After all, he feels by making this concession, he is honoring the notion of being a man that he was taught. But at the same time a man may brood, feeling like his own needs really go unmet. He may have difficulty seeing that his needs and opinions still matter, even if they are not in agreement with his romantic partner's. In this situation, there's no doubt that the line about being responsible for others becomes very blurred.

## RELATIONSHIP RED ZONE:
### Types of Empathic Failures

Below is a summary of the specific types of empathic failures relating to boys and men. To help keep these different versions in mind, let's use the acronym BACK. Remember: "Empathic failures will break a man's BACK." I know this is cheesy, but it will help you remember the concept better.

B = Empathic failures due to boundary violations (These failures can involve parents grooming a son to become an emotional partner.)

A = Empathic failures by not seeing or valuing the authentic aspects of who he is as a man (This type of failure involves devaluing or simply not appreciating his unique version of being his own man.)

C = Empathic failures in moments of vulnerability or crisis (These can involve being distracted, uncomfortable, or clumsy with tending to someone when they show vulnerability.)

K = Not keeping unresolved issues in check (These involve a parent or partner's unresolved issues related to men and masculinity. It may include a father trying to make his son the kind of man he couldn't be, a mother telling her son that men are corrupt, unreliable, or hypersexual, or a partner carrying his or her own unchecked legacy of father issues into the romantic relationship.)

# V Spot Fouls

One of the conclusions you may have already drawn from this chapter is that many men are primed to react with intensity to V Spot fouls. There can be a legacy of hurt that makes the V Spot an area of extreme vulnerability and pain. When it gets stepped on, old hurts are revealed, making for potentially explosive situations. While the exact location and intensity of these points will vary, it almost always has its roots in shame and empathic failures in one or more of the ways we have looked at so far.

The results of these chronic empathic failures can be far-reaching. They can leave men feeling fragmented inside and unsure of who they really are aside from the pain they carry and the fear of someone discovering it. Or they become so geared toward pleasing someone important to them that they lose their sense of identity. It may also leave some men with an unclear sense about boundaries, not entirely sure who is responsible for what, to whom, and to what degree. These ongoing troubles tap men's reservoirs of emotional resources, causing them to be spread thin and prone to surliness or depression.

When you hit a V Spot, you may see a man react in angry ways. He may utilize flamethrower rage and aim it at the perceived perpetrator. He may yell, rant and rave, or angrily make tracks for the door. Or he may quietly smolder. You know something is wrong, but he has closed down all entryways to keep you from actually talking about it. You may just get mean looks across the dinner table.

V Spot reactions can also include when a man takes that same flamethrower rage and points it at himself. The lessons of shame in his man-training have taught him to feel worthless in the face of perceived accusations and shortcomings. He is picking up right where he left off as a child. He believes himself insignificant and unworthy of love and may react in ways that are very self-destructive, confirming in his own mind how worthless he really is. Some men go on binges of self-pity, alcohol, drugs, or porn.

The intensity of V Spot material tells us something about the degree of hurt a man can carry inside. If he shows all that intensity to the outside world, you can bet it is at least matched to the same degree in his inner world as well. The rule of thumb is that the more intensity, the greater the damaged parts. For some men the V Spot is localized to one aspect of their lives, while for others, the V Spot has the expansive properties of global warming, where the dimensions of his pain seem to cover the entire surface of his being.

I once led a men's support group in which there was a continuum of men with various levels of emotional and psychological health. There were group members who were relatively high-functioning and well-adjusted but had areas they wanted to fine-tune regarding their manhood. Sometimes this involved making peace with a parent or re-sorting specific messages they were told about being a man. Many of these men were already well on their way to becoming their own men before they entered the group. They wanted to continue to work in the midst of relatively successful lives.

There were other group members who were experiencing a deeper sense of trouble. Many of these men could have easily fit into support groups for depression and anxiety, and some were even candidates for more intense types of psychiatric services. While each man had a different task to accomplish, what was common to them all was how their notion of being a man—and how to define that—was core to their identities.

It is important to learn more about the pain that instigates a man's V Spot wound, because it will help you get a clearer picture of his internal world as you begin to build true empathy and understanding for him. He usually already has a legacy of empathic failures under his belt. In some cases, more damage to the V Spot has occurred in the areas of adult relationships, both romantic and otherwise, especially when they have been disappointing and harmful.

If you are his partner, wife, family member, or friend and have experienced a V Spot explosion, you may think you are responsible, but chances are the intensity did not originate with you, nor was it exclusive to this singular interaction. It is actually a cumulative effect. It's helpful to look at some specific ways that V Spots get activated in the present and also how they are attached to prior shame assaults and empathic failures from the past.

This is not an exhaustive list, but in each instance we will look at how a specific type of empathic failure often results in the formation of a particular V Spot wound. While this may not be 100 percent comprehensive in every case, it will provide a starting place to help build your level of understanding and empathy. So look for the "V Spot Profile" in each section. By knowing the ins and outs of his vulnerable spots, you will not only increase your understanding of the man you love, you may also be able to bring healing to these troubled areas.

# Never Living Up to Daddy

There is a special relationship between a father and his daughter. Each captures the other's heart in a way that is beyond words. You can see this throughout their relationship, starting at the birth, where stoic men who don't show their emotions turn to jelly. Of course, there is also the stereotype of the overprotective father who screens all of her dates and quietly threatens would-be suitors' early demise if they harm her in any way. Many fathers enjoy the close bond with their "little girls" even when they are grown up.

While women may base their blueprint of an ideal man in part upon their fathers, their eventual romantic partner will not be able to measure up to Daddy. The would-be partner is at a disadvantage because he is probably younger and not as well established financially or emotionally. But the biggest difference is the nature of the father/daughter relationship. It is the father's job to tend to the daughter's needs, to be Big Daddy and take care of her; there is not an expected reciprocity.

This can be problematic when a daughter makes this lopsided blueprint the standard for finding her ideal man, desiring to feel taken care of in an unrealistic way. There may be a lingering hope that the same level of one-sided care she experienced with her father will be what she experiences in her adult romantic relationships. Those who believe this may be in for a rude awakening.

For some men, it is very troubling to never measure up to their fathers-in-law. While this may occur in many areas, it is the emotional one that causes the most harm. This can be especially true when there is ongoing conflict between the father and the husband. It is like a tug-of-war over the same woman. The daughter/wife feels stuck in the middle, trying not to offend either man she loves.

But it is the nature of growing up that while she always holds her father dear, he must play second fiddle to her husband. To not make that transition leaves a romantic relationship on shaky ground, as it sends an unspoken message that her husband is not her man. A man needs to know that his wife has successfully made the switch from daughter to wife, and when push comes to shove, the couple takes priority. When it does not, a man may feel like his wife sides against him in favor of her father. "Oh, that is not true," she may say. "You just don't understand my dad like I do." That may be true, but her husband's V Spot gets stepped on nonetheless. This type of situation begins to build resentments and intensifies the competition for loyalty.

In this delicate situation, where the daughter does not make the emotional leap to wife, the man will feel compelled to step up and redraw new boundaries with his in-laws in the hope this will change things. For example, the husband may make comments regarding the duration or frequency of in-law visits; or he may feel the need to set his father-in-law straight as to who is in charge in his marriage and home.

This may even find its way into child-rearing issues, with the husband saying something like this to his father-in-law, "You did a fine job parenting, but my wife and I are in charge of raising our own kids, so please abide by our rules for child rearing." As you can imagine, there may be huffing and puffing when these stands are taken. The message is clear that, while valuing the in-law ties, the couple has formed their own family. And this is yet another chance for the woman to make the transition from daughter to wife by supporting her husband. In these moments, it is like he is looking to her and saying, "Are you with me?" If she instead caves and sides with Daddy, or undermines the priority of the couple, she steps hard on her husband's V Spot.

## V Spot Profile

Some men may be more reactive to this type of situation than others. There may be a history of empathic failures, including boundary issues, in his own family. While he may not vocalize it, he may be thinking, "This feels awfully familiar in some way; boundaries were not all that clear when I was growing up either." Revisiting this same issue now in his family of choosing may stir up these old, unresolved troubles.

The boundary issue may be evident in the scenario described above: a father-in-law who crosses the line in terms of not letting go of his daughter and a daughter who has not transitioned into a wife. These are real issues. But the man is not free from responsibility either. While this is a difficult situation for anyone, it cuts particularly deep for him. Often it is the intensity of mixing old hurts with new ones that derails his ability to clearly negotiate the boundaries with in-laws in a more appropriate fashion. Instead, he may direct intense anger toward his in-laws and his romantic partner.

# Vulnerability

Some men receive mixed messages about what women want from them. For example, you may tell him to open up more and be vulnerable. When he does, however, you may react negatively. As mentioned earlier, some people are not comfortable with seeing others' pain, and it causes them to be a bit awkward in handling such situations. Other times, a negative reaction to a man acting vulnerable occurs because it is not in keeping with what you have been taught about how a "real man" behaves. Handling this in an awkward way conveys the message to him that real men don't have much pain, or if they do, they don't show it. A negative reaction in these types of situations can be experienced by a man as shame.

Besides the seemingly contradictory message of inviting a man to open up and then reacting adversely when he does, some couples also get into the pattern that there should be one person who is emotional and one who is stoic. Because this comes very close to traditional man-training, men often find themselves on the side of being the emotional rock.

However, this pattern becomes problematic when it is a one-sided situation and the role of rock belongs exclusively to one partner. In this case, the man is supposed to be the strong one, enabling his partner room to be emotional in the midst of the situation while still feeling grounded by his stoic stance. When he is not the rock, it makes the other person nervous because they have an unspoken (and often unconscious) contract in terms of their emotional roles in the relationship. Partners in these moments may find themselves very angry at their significant others without knowing exactly why: "Hey, stop that; you are supposed to be the rock! You're supposed to be the man! You are making me nervous because you're telling me you're nervous too!"

Some men may respond to this type of situation like this: "I thought you wanted me to be more open about who I am. I thought that meant we would change roles sometimes. It is hard to be the rock all the time, especially on my own bad days." These words often go unspoken because it can feel emotionally castrating to admit them. So the man sucks it up and deadens himself to his own worries so he can be the rock for yours.

## V Spot Profile

This type of pattern is related to boundary issues in the form of empathic failures. What to look for is a prior history of not having someone tend to his emotional needs as a kid. Instead, he had to always be the strong one. It may also be related to one of his caregivers inviting him to be an emotional partner or best friend instead of a son. His job description as a son was not to be his own man, but rather to take care of others to his own detriment. He felt like he was not supposed to have his own needs.

# Not Honoring His Choice of What It Means to Be a Man

A surefire way to hit the V Spot for some men is by saying these words: "Men don't do that!" It doesn't matter what he just did, said, or hinted at, you have just handed him his genitals in a doggy bag. This can be a very big empathic failure because you have just devalued his notion of what it means to be a man. What happens in this process is that he recalls his prior man-training and how shame tells him what not to share with others. He thinks, "Well, I won't be mentioning that again."

An even bigger problem arises here because he assimilates the message that truly being his own man is unacceptable. This is emotionally damaging, and it teaches him not to trust his own internal compass for what he knows to be right for himself. Longer-term ramifications include learning to be out of touch with what he feels as a way of buffering against the push-pull effect of staying true to his own course versus pleasing the important others in his life.

## V Spot Profile

This history of empathic failures is related to authenticity issues and prior relationships where important others did not keep either their biases or own unsorted issues in check. It may be the case that important others had a particular agenda concerning him being the *right* kind of man. He is revisiting that issue now when he tells you who he really is, hoping it will meet your approval and acceptance. But instead, that hope is dashed by a familiar letdown, just as in the past. He feels like he is not appreciated or accepted for being who he really is. He buries his true self from view.

# Comparing Him to Other Men

For some men, the V Spot is about feeling compared to other men, those who came before or those in her present circle. He might hear this as an insult by feeling as if he does not measure up to your hopes and standards. This may range from penis size, to financial portfolio, to emotional intelligence. Some partners may say, "Men are so touchy about that sort of thing. I can't say anything in front of him. I have to censor what I say." Without being properly alerted to the deeper issues at work, it is hard not to reach that conclusion.

## V Spot Profile

The potential empathic failure has to do with keeping hopes and dreams in check. His part in this situation is that you can bet this is not the first time he has heard from someone important to him that he is not up to snuff. Sometimes comparing him to others can reactivate that old wound. He may carry the fantasy that you settled for him or that he is not enough when he hears you make comparisons to others. The reality of any relationship is that the person you love will never be the absolute complete package. There will be things about each other that you hoped for but did not get. A mark of a very solid relationship is being able to share these points with one another in a way that is open and honest without inflicting hurt. It is about talking frankly regarding each other's strengths and limitations while still confirming a commitment and love for each other. This can transition the relationship to a deeper level because all the cards are on the table and no one is leaving. Imagine a relationship where you know each other that well and feel loved and accepted.

# Tough Enough

Men have varying degrees of what we stereotypically consider *toughness*. This is usually associated with physical aspects like strength, endurance, body shape, or level of fitness. For some men, no matter how hard they try, this is not an area where they excel. While caring partners, wives, and associates may wish to toughen up their man, he knows deep down it will only go so far.

## V Spot Profile

He may hear well-intended messages from loved ones about needing to join a health club, lose weight, or learn a new sport. However, based on his own legacy, he may hear another embedded message: that in the eyes of those he loves, he is not tough enough. He may feel compelled to respond to this challenge and attempt to win the loved ones' approval or respect by undertaking one of these tough endeavors. But deep inside, he also feels the sting of an old V Spot related to authenticity wounds and/or the recollection of important others from the past not keeping their biases for him in check. He may revisit old, festering wounds in these moments, realizing his limitations in the physical arena. He needs to know that you believe he is man enough—just as he is.

# The Legacy of V Spot Fouls

In the big picture, V Spot fouls are shaped by the stringent and unforgiving Ten Commandments of Growing Up Male. Sure, men are taught these rules for how they should be and sometimes suffer for it, but these messages don't fall upon women's deaf ears either. Women pick up on the man-training, and in many cases, easily see through some of the ridiculous aspects—but not all of them.

You see, both men and women are duped by these things. They assume that some of the man-training is based in truth. I can remember very clearly having a conversation with a worldly, educated woman who asked me what I did for a living. When I told her about my work with men, she seemed a little confused, saying, "Well, men don't need to talk about things, do they?" The same notion can be said for men's perceptions of themselves; they don't really recognize there is complexity and depth within because no one expects it from them.

So when a friend, partner, or family member commits a V Spot foul, it can carry an extra sting. Some men expect the world to be unsympathetic in this regard, but not those they love. Most men have their own stories to tell about these occurrences and carry the fantasy that they will one day find a safe haven to just be themselves, free of pretense or false manly posturing. Men hope that those they love, whether a romantic partner, family member, or friend, can see through all the bologna associated with being a man and not add to it.

# Making Amends

Finally, some parents, partners, or friends who read this chapter may find themselves feeling anxious. They wonder if unwittingly they have empathically failed a man they love. They may recognize themselves in this chapter in terms of how they have handled things with their sons, friends, or partners. What can be done?

First, it is helpful to confirm that these empathic failures have indeed occurred. This often begins with a realistic appraisal of past situations. If you realize you've failed your man, it is normal to experience a certain amount of guilt. But remember that even well-intended people have areas in which they need to grow, and learning the subtle nuances of being empathically attuned to another is hard work.

Also, please don't speak to your son, husband, partner, or friend in a way that is aimed at alleviating your own sense of remorse. Do not go to him and say, "I read in this book about empathic failures and men and how damaging that can be, and I know I have never failed you in that way. Right? Right?" Instead you should work on the areas in which you need to grow as a parent, partner, or spouse in a way that will facilitate reconnection and healing.

The degree to which the other person has felt let down will determine how much reparative work needs to be done in order to make it right. There may be a period of anger and sadness that has to be tolerated. In some cases, professional help is needed to mend the relationship. Trying to make amends and beginning to relate in a different way may be very difficult at first, but it can pay off in big dividends in the relationship. It ushers in an authenticity and connection where both parties benefit. The suggestions on making amends that are given below may help.

## RELATIONSHIP RED ZONE:
### Making Amends

Making amends requires a sincere heart that admits the harm that has been done. While there are usually two sides to any story, it is important to own and make amends for your part. This process is most effective when a person is truly remorseful, verbalizes the wrong, and takes steps to right the transgression. This may include a promise not to repeat the hurtful behavior in the future or a symbolic gesture to say you're sorry.

Making amends can fail if any of these important aspects are missing. For instance, verbalizing apologies without real sincerity sabotages the whole exercise. Also, amending actions that are done begrudgingly or without real effort can destroy the amends and put the relationship in deeper trouble.

## Important Steps for Making Amends:
1. Own the harm that has been done.
2. Be sincere when making amends.
3. Take action to show that making amends is a priority.

## ▶ Toolbox Tip: Plan Your Amends Making

Sometimes finding the right words for saying you're sorry is difficult. What you mean to say may not come across exactly like you hoped in the moment. You may find yourself feeling like you are only causing more harm to an already bad situation. In the heat of the moment you may feel sincerely sorry, but at the same time, you may harbor resentment or mixed feelings for having to make amends: "Why doesn't he make amends first for what he has done? Why is it that I have to always say sorry first?!" You may have to clear your own plate first so you can make amends with a sincere heart. If you feel like you can't do it without slipping into a resentful mode, you may want to plan your amends on paper. The plan below could be a helpful guide.

1. Make your heart as ready as you can to make amends. You may have to mentally picture how you have hurt the one you love. Imagine in your mind's eye how it must feel to be on the other end of the wrong. You have to draw on your best empathic attunement skills here. As you ramp up to make amends, you may need to come back to this place of empathy throughout the day to stay out of the resentful mode.

2. Write down what you want to say ahead of time. This may take several drafts. Go back and look through what you wrote, letting your sincerity be your guide. The key is to make sure you don't put any little barbs in there because you are still mad. You may get a trusted friend to proof what you wrote.

3. Select a quiet time to actually deliver the amends. Nothing is worse than trying to open up during a difficult situation and having your family member, friend, or partner say, "I didn't hear you; what did you say?" Of course, it can make matters worse if you feel like he is being gamey by not hearing, "Well . . . I said I was sorry, but if you didn't hear it the first time, tough, loser."

4. Read aloud what you wrote and put yourself into what you say. You might be surprised how emotional it may feel when saying the words in the other person's presence versus the rehearsals.

5. Don't expect instant miracles. Realize that, depending on the depth of hurt, it may not only take time for the amends to sink in, but it also might involve showing signs of new behavior in old situations. You can also ask, "Is there anything I can do to make this better?"

# Conclusion

We have learned that empathic failures can occur when parents, partners, or friends are out of sync with what is needed in moments of vulnerability or crisis. They can also occur when men are put down for just being themselves or are forced to deal with inappropriate boundary situations. Sometimes empathic failures occur just because it is hard to think or feel oneself into another's inner world, which is further complicated by a legacy of hurts from the past. It can make it hard to know how to respond.

When empathic failures occur on a chronic basis, long-standing and negative psychological consequences may result. Individuals who have experienced such treatment have a general sense of feeling fragmented inside, and they lack the emotional resources to deal effectively with life's demands. These types of chronic empathic failures are the core experiences related to a broken or fragile sense of personhood.

Now for the really hard part for romantic partners out there: remember No. 7 and No. 8 of the Ten Commandments of Growing Up Male: "If your father is rejecting, you must learn to please him" and "If you don't please your mother, you must marry someone like her." These two commandments can be the original source of much of the V Spot damage. They also may have influenced how he chose a mate. Depending on how much healing he has done regarding these earliest relationships, he may still feel compelled to revisit some of these old conflicts in later relationships in the hopes that another pass will lead to a different outcome. That is, he may have unwittingly picked someone as a romantic partner who emotionally resembles a parent with whom he has V Spot issues.

In the best-case scenario, a man will find someone who knows what he needs and will commit to meeting those needs. If you are a partner and reading this book, you might be thinking, "Well, my partner or husband did that when he chose me. I know exactly what to say and do." I hate to be the bearer of bad news, but that may not be entirely true. If you placed someone (male or female) in a roomful of potential mates who are ready and willing to give them what they need, they will often feel magnetically drawn to the one soul hidden in the corner who in some way resembles what they experienced when growing up.

It may sound crazy that they would pick such a person when there are so many others who are ready and able to give them what they need, but there is something about working through old hurts that takes priority. The Latin phrase *similia similibus curantur*, which means "like is cured by like," expresses how old emotional wounds are healed. Depending on his history of V Spot wounds and his current level of working through them, he may pick someone who has *some* qualities similar to those of a hurtful parent from his past.

Now, after you have braced yourself, had a quick drink, or thrown this book against the wall in frustration or disbelief, there is some good news. Just as he has V Spots and has chosen someone who will hopefully help him recover from them, there is a reason you chose him as well. Again, depending on your own history, you may have picked him in part to help heal your own wounds. He is probably similar to one or both of your parents in some good and not-so-good ways.

You and he are a hand-in-glove fit for each other. You chose each other with the hope of finding healing and peace. If you are mindful and committed to doing that, then both of you will benefit. Get to know his V Spots and let him know yours. The love and intention to purposefully help each other—being guardians for each other—allows the past hurts to heal. There is no greater gift than growing for yourself and the one you love.

# CHAPTER CUES

1. V Spots are men's extreme places of vulnerability and wounding.

2. The intensity of reactions to V Spot fouls reflects the severity of the wounds that created them.

3. V Spots are formed through shame and empathic failures.

4. Remember the acronym BACK to recall the different types of empathic failures.

5. V Spots are healed through empathy and understanding.

6. Often both men and women unconsciously seek out romantic partners who are like caregivers in both healthy and not-so-healthy ways.

7. In a romantic relationship, helping mend each other's V Spots deepens the connection.

# 10

## How to Offer Constructive Feedback to a Man

As a clinician, I can recall a number of times when I asked a male psychotherapy client, "Are there any issues you need to talk about? Or any issues specifically related to being a man we should address?" and he'd stare back blankly and answer, "No." Sometimes I know this is just the initial difficulty of being in therapy; it isn't easy for anyone. Sometimes making it to the door of my office is a challenge in itself.

I remember one man who spoke with me on the phone for a good five minutes, trying repeatedly to find the right words for saying he would like to set up an appointment. It had all the heightened anxiety and potential pain of rejection that went along with asking someone out on a first date. With all this in mind, there are still circumstances when a man is a bit clueless—not only about the issues he faces, but also about how the repercussions of his actions affect himself or others; these issues simply do not register in any significant way on his personal radar.

For some of these men, issues from the past still haunt them. Certainly some of their experiences have been very damaging, involving shame, ridicule, or even physical abuse for not "being a man." Others are told by their wives that unless they seek help, the relationship is over, because she and the children are nervous and uncomfortable in their presence. Still others may hear from their bosses that they really need to speak to someone about all the anger they misplace onto fellow employees. Given all this potential pain and suffering, it may seem odd they are unaware of their own dilemma. It is as if these aspects of themselves are not part of their conscious awareness, though those around them can see them quite clearly.

What is lacking in the situations described above is the ability of a man to psychologically step away and observe himself in an objective fashion. To be able to do this is a mark of healthy emotional development. It is like having a "man cam" where someone videotaped his actions throughout the day so he could then go back and review them. He could evaluate how he interacted with his boss, wife, children, or friends.

These "tapes" are important because they have high-definition clarity; they are not blurred with preconceived conclusions, anger, or disappointment. He can consider the events of the day and get an accurate read about what really happened. He can make use of feedback concerning missteps, or other times, rightfully utilize the man cam to support his actions. Reviewing the episodes of the day allows him to gain an objective perspective on his thoughts, feelings, and behavior.

But the man cam extends its usefulness beyond events that happened today. It can also provide a retrospective picture of a person's life, including a sense of how his definition of being a man has evolved. It can show his strengths as well as those aspects of his masculinity that still need sorting out. This includes being able to approach those situations in the archives of his life when he fell short and facing them squarely without resorting to blurring the past.

He also makes note of past triumphs, celebrating moments when his own authentic way of being really emerged. He can build upon all these events in order to construct his signature version of being himself. Having the man cam on also enables him to accurately perceive individuals and events that had an influence on him, for good or bad. It will both aid in making peace with his shadow parents and help him recollect those who rendered assistance. To make the best use of all the information mentioned above, it needs to be on the radar screen of personal awareness. Otherwise, a man cannot learn from the past or move forward in his life with any real certainty.

When the man cam is operative from his formative years onward, a man learns to see himself the way others see him; they act as a mirror that reflects his behavior back to him and are able to give accurate feedback. When men are valued for who they really are, they sense that spirit of affirmation even in the midst of constructive feedback. The degree to which a man is able to receive these types of important experiences (seeing and valuing) will determine the clarity of the lens for his man cam. For some men, the lens cover is still on the man cam because they received skewed feedback in their formative years and were never appreciated for who they genuinely were; others' man cams will show certain distortions or be a little out of focus.

## The Man Cam and the Potential to Take in Feedback

Developing the man cam occurs slowly over time, but it is a necessary skill for a good life. While having an honest appraisal of oneself is important in its own right, it also builds the foundation for receiving constructive feedback, which in turn gives males of all ages the potential for growth. Sometimes feedback can indicate that something he is doing comes across as edgy, or possibly pushes others away, even those he cares about. Even thoughtful, kindhearted men are often not aware of all aspects of their interactions and what impact they have on themselves and others. In these situations, feedback from others can be corrective because it allows a man to see and respond to areas in need of growth.

All of us receive feedback constantly—from our surroundings, the people in our lives, even the sensations in our own bodies—but the Ten Commandments of Growing Up Male teach men to turn down the volume on this information if it will lead to potential conflict about what it means to be a man. In other cases, especially in the formative years, men have listened too well to feedback from others and have come away feeling deeply wounded. It may feel as if who they are is being questioned. The ultimate fear is that they might not measure up as a man.

Because men often experience feedback as a potentially corrupting and devastating force, they quickly learn to protect themselves by turning a deaf ear to others. This is a psychological defense misconstrued by some as a sturdy, go-it-alone attitude; others view it as having the gumption to stick to your guns. What men need to do instead is not only turn up the volume on the feedback but learn to evaluate the credibility of the information. It is by developing mastery over the volume switch, as well as increasing keenness and clarity of perception, that he most effectively utilizes the man cam. When he can see himself through the eyes of others, considering and weighing the merit of the feedback, over time he will learn how to objectively assess what is being conveyed.

As mentioned above, one of the key reasons feedback gets short-circuited is because it can feel terribly threatening. Discussions that concern whether or not he is being "man enough" can be emotionally laden. Although not all attempts at feedback are initially directed at his sense of being a man, many nonetheless find their way there. Sooner or later, all rivers flow to that ocean.

Sometimes the sense of masculinity is in the foreground of the situation, and in these cases, aspects of masculinity are explicitly discussed. Many men know these types of conversations, where they are instructed on appropriate manly behavior or admonished for breaking proper protocol regarding the Commandments. Other times, masculinity is in the background, acting as the long, complex thread that ties together every aspect of a man's life across his many different roles: son, father, friend, partner, brother, lover, and so on.

Whether in the foreground or background, being a man is the one constant across all other identities in his life. It can be an omnipresent force within a man's psyche, constantly posing the question, "Did I measure up as a man?" in each role. It is the reason partners sometimes get a bit confused when men become overly defensive about unsolicited instructions on how to mow the lawn or bristle when feedback is less than stellar, at least in their perception. Sooner or later, it all comes into contact with that core part of his person: being a man. It is a socially engineered way to construct the foundation of his identity. For those men whose sense of masculinity is fraught with unresolved issues, its all-pervasive status means coming into contact with conflict/pain on a daily basis; for these men, their sense of masculinity is a liability, a constant drain on their resources at each turn of their lives.

But imagine a different scenario, one in which the sense of masculinity, the common tie that binds all his responsibilities and endeavors, is at peace and old conflicts are sorted out. In this case, he has a clear notion of who he is and how he wants to live. A man's sense of masculinity becomes a rich resource, bolstering who he is every step of the way along life's journey. The ability to receive feedback can bring this to fruition in his life. Feedback promotes growth in the necessary areas, allowing a man to live more comfortably in his own skin. This allows him to carve out his own notion of how to be a man. This is one of the many reasons that utilizing the man cam is so important. For many, it is the means by which they will discover a different way of living.

Eventually, with enough experience in receiving constructive feedback from others, a man can act as a source of direct feedback for himself. Men can learn what it feels like when they are off-kilter and can pay attention to the red flags. This can occur when they push others away or demand too much of people. Reflective men have learned through the feedback of others about both the verbal and nonverbal ways they show themselves when they are not at their best. This could include tone of voice, facial gestures, word choice, and so on. After having heard this feedback from others enough times, they can slowly detect within themselves when they are engaging in those behaviors. It is like looking through their man camcorder and a flashing red light appears: "Warning, warning, you are not your best self right now!" "Warning, warning, you are reenacting old conflicts with your dad and playing them out with your boss!" "Warning, warning, you are about to step over the line with your wife and are looking at a night on the sofa." The positive, healthy reaction to this feedback is for a man to take corrective steps as his own personal man cam notices and gives him feedback on what he is doing.

### ▶ Toolbox Tip: Man Cam and Feedback

Feedback, while at times uncomfortable, does not have to be feared. The man cam allows for a more neutral, even-tempered appraisal of the information being offered about him. This, in turn, allows him to consider the validity of feedback without experiencing an emotional meltdown. That is, a personal style does not necessarily have to slide into a defensive one. Or if it does, it is just a temporary misstep when the man cam comes to his aid. This allows the necessary internal adjustments, like saying to himself, "This feedback is not meant as a personal attack." Then he can relax more and engage the conversation as need be.

The man cam develops this ability to take in feedback through a personal history of guardians who "see" him and then respond to him in a way that is not damaging to his core sense of worth. That is, feedback is given about important areas of potential growth. However, feedback is not to be equated with "what's wrong with you" or "proof positive that you are a flawed man without worth." The best feedback confirms the worth of the person while pointing out areas in need of change without judgment. Of course, it is best when men have received this type of care from an early age, but for many this is something they experience and develop in their adult lives. It becomes something they learn with the assistance of their partners and peers.

# Man Defenses

Feedback goes astray when it is perceived as a threat; the knee-jerk reaction is to employ some type of defense as a means of protection. Defenses can occur in the inner and outer worlds. In both cases, defenses are meant to keep hurtful things from being experienced. In the internal realm of the psyche, defenses are an emotional shield, deflecting difficult pain or conflict that already circles around inside. We have already looked at the need to turn down the volume on feedback from others or one's own internal dialogue; these are examples of internal defenses. But there are other forms of defense as well, like rationalizing behaviors or detaching from emotions.

When defenses happen in the outer world, it is usually in the context of relating to others. For instance, a man may hear feedback as a personal attack, so he attacks back: "Well, now it is my turn to tell you what is wrong with you." He may try to place distance between himself and the author of the feedback: "I am going out for a drink with my friends." Or he may hear the feedback and quickly concede any and all points to cease the feedback immediately: "I totally agree with everything you say. Are we done now?" In each of these scenarios, feedback does not hit its mark. In order to understand defenses more, we first need to look at basic relationship skills and build from there.

As psychoanalyst Karen Horney noted, in most healthy relationships there are three necessary skills of relating: moving toward, moving away, and moving against. "Moving toward" in healthy form has to do with compromise and compliance. We make appropriate efforts to get along with those we love, realizing that in all loving relationships moments of strain are normal and par for the course. We learn we cannot always have it our way and that the basis for a lasting relationship is making peace, practicing forgiveness, and not expecting it to always be fifty/fifty in terms of give and take. When we move toward someone, we employ that giving part of ourselves, offering loving-kindness. "Moving away" deals with a sense of self-reliance and autonomy. A person draws upon their own resources to manage tasks and difficult moments when needed. Even in genuine, loving connections, we are not really joined at the hip and are called to act independently. Sometime this "me time" also helps us get back in touch with the authentic sense of who we are. Finally, "moving against" involves being aware of what one needs and voicing it; at heart it is the assertive quality to stand one's ground, even in conflicted moments with loved ones. Enduring and embracing these moments is important, as they clear the air in a relationship. When necessary, the moving against action can also reset relationship patterns that are not working. These conversations often begin with, "I need to speak with you for a few moments about something . . ." Moving against is a healthy part of pruning the thorns in connections with others.

Each of these skills is vital for possessing a healthy sense of oneself and being with others. There is also a natural fluidity, as one ebbs and flows, using these various abilities when the situation calls for it. We can think of these skills as part of the natural rhythm of any relationship. Let's refer to it as the "ebb and flow cycle of intimacy." For instance, there are times couples go through periods when they are in perfect sync with each other. The stereotypical example is when each member of a couple may move toward one another at the same time. This usually results in a sense of harmony, connection, or even romance.

Likewise, the traditional place of complaint in the cycle is when one partner moves away and the other moves toward. For instance, one person may need time to themselves after a hard day, and the other is ready for some couple time. This lack of being in sync can promote both conscious and unconscious reactions on the part of each partner that range from feeling smothered to feeling abandoned. Each partner may wonder, in various ways, "Don't they know what I need right now? Why are they so unwilling to give it?" This can result in feeling hurt, angry, or deserted.

Given our individual histories, it is normal that each of us feels more comfortable using some skills more than others; this explains why we can be at different points in the ebb and flow cycle of intimacy. These points are where communication is most likely to break down. In certain parts of the relationship cycle (moving toward, away from, or against), some people get stuck, in part because there is a lack of clear communication and understanding of underlying motives. While ill intent may be read into these situations, what may actually be happening is that each person is just at a different place in terms of their needs. The trick is being able to recognize that the ebb and flow is a part of the natural order of relationships and not a means of hurting each other. Most important for each member of the couple is realizing that a viable and deep connection can be maintained across all aspects of the ebb and flow cycle of intimacy; it just takes time to develop a sense of trust in the relationship and one another. This will assure some that being intimate does not have to result in being emotionally smothered. Likewise, there are ways to enjoy being separate, healthy individuals while still maintaining the sense of being a couple.

Adding to communication challenges is that one or both people in a couple may not know how to avoid a relationship rut, or, once in, they may struggle to get out. Most partners have some sense of what these points of disconnection look like: everything is fine, but don't expect him or her to let you be too close for too long. Or when he is in a bad place, he goes off to his cave until he is ready to come out. Or he is a very easygoing person, but if you cross him, watch out—he has a bad temper. Or he lets things build up inside and never tells you when he is upset. To get back on track successfully takes mastering the basic aspects of each of the intimacy cycle skills. Taken together, preferences, as well as areas that need honing, become the basis for forming a personality style that governs our interactions with others.

While each of the skills above may be employed at some point and under certain circumstances, chances are a man (or a woman) will have a predominant style based on moving toward, moving against, or moving away from others. This is their usual way of dealing with others in normal, everyday living. The real challenge—and what helps us understand more about communication and giving feedback—is having an accurate perception of these strengths and limitations.

We should be aware of the potential places in the ebb and flow intimacy cycle where a person is most likely to become derailed. It is also important to realize that, under stress, each person's predominant style can do a dysfunctional slide, given the right circumstances. That is, his biggest strengths under regular conditions can become a liability under duress. This slide into a defensive posture often happens when a person or a relationship is under a significant amount of situational or chronic strain; in these cases, a man's default setting in personal style can emerge in dysfunctional ways. The result is an inflexible stance, one that often prohibits other needed skills from coming into play. This is another key reason people become stuck in the ebb and flow intimacy cycle.

Let's look at the specific ways each of these styles can be functional in everyday living, but dysfunctional in stressful circumstances, often causing communication difficulties, among other things.

## ▶ Toolbox Tip: Ebb and Flow in the Relationship Is the Natural Order

We have to realize that a relationship never really stays put in one place for very long. The natural tendency of relationships includes fluidity and change. This is because the two people involved are also constantly making adjustments in both their inner and outer worlds. They respond to the demands placed on them by work, kids, and other relationships.

Sometimes, the two people are in perfect sync in the cycle, resulting in a blissful harmony. At this point, couples really remember why they got into the relationship in the first place. All the other stuff seems to fade from memory. Sometimes the couple may think this state of being in perfect sync is a permanent achievement. Some will take this as a sign that the relationship is finally on the right track, but in reality, just as the people involved make adjustments, so does the relationship. There will be times in the cycle when closeness is at a premium and other times when feeling separate is just a normal reaction to what is going on.

The "moving toward" style appears in its most functional form in a man who is emotionally available and has the potential to open up and even be vulnerable. He seems present and wanting to connect, willing to share his inner world and wanting to know about yours. He is ready to make compromises and seems easygoing about decision making. Many would describe him as the prototypical "nice guy" who will put up with a host of unpleasant things without complaint: "Wow, that Charlie is a real saint." However, when this style is under a significant amount of stress, compromise in a relationship can quickly become appeasement. In worst-case situations, he may idealize his significant other(s) (friend, partner, or boss), not seeing their flaws and wanting to be on their good side, as though all the decision-making power rests with them. Being seen as unselfish and good are his top priorities, not making his real needs known, even to his own detriment. The wish to connect can turn clingy and demanding. He may seem somewhat sulky when he does not have his needs met, attempting to vie for your attention and feeling slighted when he does not receive it. He may feel like he is being abandoned to his own devices but feels either too saintly or too much like a martyr to really complain. Instead, he often just stuffs his frustration inside.

For those who are particularly good at engaging others through showing their vulnerable side, there is a proneness to garner reactions of pity. "Poor guy! As they say, nice guys really do finish last." Feedback to this type of aggregated style can lack a genuine response; his top priority is ending the conflict, not having an honest conversation, even when that is what is desperately needed. Sometimes, when this type of man does accept the feedback, it seems so personalized that one feels guilty or remorseful for making it such a big deal and "hurting" him. In long-term relationships, a lack of respect for the man can be an undoing of the connection.

The "moving away" style characterizes the stereotypical self-reliant man. He really seems like he can handle most, if not all, of life's situations on his own. He is a "go-it-alone guy." He may have a certain stability and predictability about him that many find appealing. Because he seems so proficient in handling things by himself, he may also be seen as an astute man who can be relied on because of his thoughtfulness and wisdom. Viewed as the strong, silent type, and keeping his cards pretty close to the vest, many feel privileged when he allows them to help in any small way. For him, these moments of letting people in seem like monumental leaps of trust.

However, under duress, the moving away man really packs up and heads out. Self-sufficiency turns to aloofness. He may seem emotionally distant, and others may experience him as though he is behind a wall. Attempts, and sometimes pleas, are made for him to come back, at least within earshot, often to no avail; it seems these gestures of reaching out drive him further away. Many friends and romantic partners feel helpless trying to connect with him when he really moves away. Giving feedback to a man with this style can feel like tossing notes over a wall—you are not quite able to connect face to face. Sometimes they wonder if he really needs or even loves them; if so, why could he so easily separate to such a degree?

The "moving against" style man appears in his functional form as the confident person who knows what he wants and how to get it. He may have clear direction for his life and can chart his achievements from point A to point B; basically, he's unstoppable. He is usually good on his feet, fielding questions and comments with a degree of ease that makes others see him as a credible source. He can be a hero to some, showing signs of leadership and strength. He asserts his wishes and needs; one never has to guess about these matters.

But under duress, the moving against style man can become intimidating and aggressive. He will be in your face, refusing to concede points as though his life depends on it. He will appear defensive and overbearing, often dismissive of other opinions when they do not align with his own. In some situations, he can be a name-caller or a yeller, reminding you of how your offensive actions are similar to those who have hurt him before. In extreme versions, aggression in forms of physical or emotional abuse occurs. Partners and friends feel emotionally beat up in encounters with someone who moves against in intense ways. While his charm may reappear after morphing back to his normal self, some feel like they will be in for a real battle if they have to give feedback to this type of man. If there are repeated episodes of intense moving against behaviors, it begins to wear down the potential safety of the relationship. They may also come to see that it is not worth all the hassle just to talk, and avoidance of the situation or person begins to occur.

In all of the styles and corresponding defenses, there are potential benefits and liabilities. There is no "right" style. While one may have a predominant default setting, it is helpful to have the other two skill sets readily available. Having these may allow for more flexibility in everyday living and under stress, which also has an impact on receiving feedback without it getting sidetracked or misplaced. Styles become dysfunctional when they turn into rigid defenses, replacing what can be a very engaging and adaptive personal way of being; the differences between the two—style versus defense—can be aggravated by a particularly stressful single episode, or by the wearing away bit by bit over time in chronic difficulties.

## ▶ Toolbox Tip: The Style Slide

In this diagram, we can see how the basic relational skills (moving toward, away, and against) are the foundation for the development of a predominant personality style that under duress can produce a particular type of defense:

Skill    ⟶    Style    ⟶    Defense

### Relationship Red Zone: Man Defenses During Feedback

| TYPES OF STYLE | WHAT IT LOOKS LIKE |
| --- | --- |
| 1. Moves toward you | Takes the feedback too much to heart, premature appeasement, fears abandonment |
| 2. Moves away from you | Emotionally distant; goes blank or shuts down; physically removes himself; takes a walk or goes for a beer with friends |
| 3. Moves against you | Compares you to other hurtful people in his life; makes accusations and bears his teeth |

# Understanding Man Defenses

It will help enormously in your attempts to communicate with your man in sticky moments if you can see beyond the surface when a style slide activating the man defenses has occurred. This involves perceiving what is really going on and not getting hooked by appearances. First, realize that defenses are employed to protect vulnerable areas in the heart and mind; they are a temporary shield for old wounds and are aggravated when others pass near in the process of communicating feedback.

As mentioned in previous chapters, this is where the world of shadow parents fogs the clear perception of actual events. Old snippets from well-worn family dramas may begin playing in his mind, specifically those related to being a man or not measuring up. He may feel himself regress in power and maturity. He may become nervous, fearful, or even aggressive, trying to ward off those who come too close. Because he may have tunnel vision in these moments, he may confuse you with those from his past, trying to figure out if you are friend or foe. So be aware that you are going into a potentially murky arena where the past and present collide—all the more reason to proceed with caution and a clear head.

Also, making note of the level of intensity he seems to experience when you try to give him feedback will help you know if this is one of those areas that needs special consideration, representing a V Spot for him. Remember, the telltale sign of old wounds is emotional intensity: the more intense the reaction, the deeper the level of emotional damage it represents. When he goes off the Richter scale, it's usually a sign that a deeper nerve has been struck. In this case, tread carefully and convey that your communication is not meant to pick up where someone else left off; verbalizing that point and using your empathy skills is helpful: "Look, I know you have been hurt by others in the past, but that is not my intention here." In fact, your purpose is the exact opposite; you want to bring order and peace to an area in his psyche that needs healing. Offering feedback in a nonthreatening way can help achieve this.

Finally, while defensiveness can be annoying, most defensive maneuvers are used to avoid getting wounded again, and this is important to keep in mind. As a man becomes more aware of his actions through the use of his man cam, it is fair game to make known to him these awkward moments when he is too [fill in the blank]. You can approach him by saying, "I want to be there for you, and it makes it easier for me to do this if you would not [fill in the blank] and perhaps do a little bit more of [fill in the blank]." Be specific in terms of what you are asking for by naming behaviors, tone of voice, gestures, and so on. It's best to have these discussions after the heat of the moment, but sometimes having them in the middle of a conflict is necessary to keep forward momentum.

While this may sound like you are making him the sole focus of communication, the ultimate aim is that you stretch for each other. This point really needs to be stressed: you are both signing up for this work together. It helps couples break dysfunctional communication styles and keeps them from going back into old patterns. This is a reciprocal way to grow both personally and within the relationship. This commitment to oneself and each other keeps things emotionally grounded, even when it is hard not to let one of those old zingers fly or when sidestepping a mean comment.

The other thing that helps is knowing the complete package of a man's defense style, which includes his strengths, liabilities, and where he is prone to be stuck in the ebb and flow cycle of intimacy. The final part involves knowing the underlying causes/personal history of his hurts and defenses. Taken together, this allows one to see a man's defensive moments with softer eyes. These are the keys to staying nonreactive and keeping constructive conversations from turning into full-blown fights.

# Giving Feedback

Giving someone feedback is a skill that includes holding the right balance of support and challenge. One tries to value and love the person even in the midst of giving needed pointers. There needs to be an underlying, unconditional care when giving feedback. The reason we give feedback is to help someone we care about, not to settle old scores through exposing and taking advantage of another's vulnerabilities. Some may read this and think, "Easier said than done." They would be quite right if the person in question seems fragile and cannot take in the feedback without resorting to the defensive maneuvers mentioned above. Those types of defensive reactions have the potential to pull a loved one off balance; they lose their stance of loving-kindness. To prevent this from happening, we need to take a more point-by-point approach.

## Feedback Pointers

1. *It is always good to be thoughtful about choosing when to give feedback.* You don't try to have this type of discussion in a noisy restaurant or when trying to put the kids to bed. You don't have it when you are pressed for time, and you certainly don't have it in the middle of an argument about something else by lobbing the feedback in impulsively. You may have wanted to talk about this for a long time and your anger may compel you to blurt it out. Or worse yet, you feel like hurting your partner and you know this topic gives you the ammunition you need to do it. Instead, you need to ask your partner if you can set aside some time to talk about something that is of concern to you: "Is now a good time to talk and could we take a few minutes to discuss something? If this is not a good time, let's put something down on the calendar for later in the day or tomorrow."

2. *The most successful way to give feedback is to adopt the attitude that you want to give it because you really do love the person and believe that what they are doing is somehow destructive to himself, you, or the relationship.* You believe that giving this feedback will somehow help him bridge the gap between his past and the present and make for a more content life. You also know that you have to put your own emotional armor on, and if your partner is someone who uses defensive maneu-

vers about feedback, you must be prepared to take an even-tempered stance and not get pulled into reacting.

3. *Just as your partner may have a signature way of maneuvering defensively, you may also have your own idiosyncratic way of responding to it that may make things worse.* For instance, men who respond to feedback by distancing may pull you into a defensive mode. You may feel hurt that he is not listening and say to yourself or out loud, "Fine—go and get a drink with your friends, you stupid jerk!" Or you may feel unloved and beg him not to go, "Stay and let's keep talking about this if you really love me!" which only makes him move out the door quicker. There can be a number of different responses that may be unhelpful. After some honest self-examination, determine what the trigger points are for you and decide you won't employ them while giving feedback. You have to be steadfast in these tenuous moments.

4. *After initially mustering up the courage to speak your mind, begin to share your feedback in a thoughtful manner.* You may want to practice what you will say beforehand; you may even write it down so you can convey your feelings in a way that is not hurtful. The thing about feedback is that most people can sense when it is coming from a place of care and concern versus an attempt to dig at someone's insecurities or frailties. Even when the contents do sting somewhat, they can sense that loving-kindness is behind it. Remember, the point of the feedback is to eventually enhance the contentment of the other person, though in the moment it may feel as though you are doing anything but that. You have to stick to your guns. Be strong in these moments, believing that what you are doing is the right thing.

5. *Be clear and specific in your feedback.* Then give the other person time to process what was said, time to react, and if need be, time to ask questions. There may be a defensive response, but in most cases this can be neutralized by trying to understand and talk through the person's reactions. Usually being patient in a nonjudgmental way and encouraging them to speak about what is going on before assessing the

validity of the feedback is often necessary. "What are you feeling now that I have given my feedback?" "You seem to be feeling angry or hurt—is that right?" Honestly, you may have to spend more time sorting out the hurt feelings that are expressed as defensive maneuvers than drilling home the actual feedback. They may make references to you being just like "so and so" (e.g., their mother or father). Instead of saying, "No I am not, you loser," you may say instead, "How does it seem that way?" making use of your emotional armor by not reacting to being compared to this person you may not like. In allowing them to air the comparisons, they may stumble upon the fact that there really are differences between you and the person you are being compared to—one being that you are steady enough to withstand some conflict in the relationship without taking it personally, and another being that you will not belittle him or abandon him when things are difficult. This type of interaction, while sometimes exhausting, may actually strengthen your relationship. The level of intimacy and trust may increase as you help remove some of the defensive maneuvers that block more honest discussion. You may even gain insight into the hurts your partner carries inside.

6. *Once the hurt feelings are out of the way, which may take some time, the feedback can be considered.* However, don't expect it to be taken in all at once. Sometimes people need time away from the discussion to mull over what was said. You may have to end the initial feedback with recognizing this is as far as it can go for now. You may give words of encouragement and care to your partner and tell them they are welcome to talk with you more when they are ready. Remember, the feedback is given because you care about this person and want them to have a better life. When they sense this is the motivation, chances are they will be more able to hear it.

7. *Be prepared to go down unexpected paths.* If you ask for this type of honest exploration, you may get more than you bargained for. You may hear things from your loved one that he has been thinking about

for some time but has not verbalized. You are giving permission for those types of things to be said. It may change the fundamental way you and he interact. By having these honest discussions, you are potentially placing old issues on the table that have been present but not talked about (the pink elephant in the room that both of you have seen but neither have acknowledged).

In addition, this may be the first time you're hearing about situations from the past that were hurtful to him. He may reveal pains from an earlier period that were confusing, difficult, and that still plague him. Perhaps the worst thing that can happen here is to move into a place of emotional reactivity and judgment. You may hear things you don't like or that make you uncomfortable. There may be a choice to sort these things out now or at a later time in order to stay on the task for the moment.

8. *The feedback has usually not run its course after the initial talk is over.* Your partner may come back and say he wants to talk more about what you discussed. Or you may wait a few days and check in to see how things are settling. You can get an update in this way, but real closure may be further down the road. It is hard to be patient in these moments, and some will be tempted to nag because things are not moving quickly enough; others might feel insecure, fearing things are really hanging in the balance. During these times, it may be best to place the discussion on the shelf as much as possible and concentrate on other things like work, exercise, and visiting with other friends. Ruminating about it too much can be harmful, because it may lead to resentment: "Stupid man! I try to help him out with his man cam, and what does he do? He doesn't even tell me what is going on . . . that's the last time I try to help him!"

▶ **Toolbox Tip: Steps for Giving Feedback**

1. Choose the correct time to give feedback.
2. Feedback should always be given in a spirit of love.
3. You have your own idiosyncratic way of giving and receiving feedback.
4. Share your feedback in a thoughtful manner.
5. Be clear and specific in your feedback.
6. Get beyond hurt feelings before considering the actual feedback.
7. Be prepared to go down unexpected paths.
8. Remember that it takes time for feedback to sink in.

## RELATIONSHIP RED ZONE:
### Rephrasing Hurtful Communications

| THE MEAN WAY | A BETTER WAY |
|---|---|
| 1. Name-calling | Identify specific behaviors that offend or hurt. |
| 2. Purposefully trying to wound him | Give feedback in the spirit of trying to make the situation better for you and the one that you love. |
| 3. Using a barrage of words that are designed to hurt him intentionally | Use honest, strong words when needed, but realize a little goes a long way. |
| 4. Holding grudges | If the relationship is going to work, some hurts have to be placed in the relationship stream to be carried away. |
| 5. Withholding love or affection in a punishing way to show him who is boss | Making up cannot only be fun, it can allow a tender, connecting feeling back into the relationship. |

# RELATIONSHIP RED ZONE:
## Map Out How Your Fights Normally Go

Below are some typical he says/she says responses that go with particular man defenses. Note how both people participate in making the situation worse. See if any of these patterns of disconnect are similar to what happens for you and your man.

## SOME TYPICAL MAN DEFENSES

### I. MOVING TOWARD STYLE

*He Says:*

"I am so sorry baby . . . I will make it up, I promise!" (grovel, grovel). "I always knew I was a worthless man, and what you said proves it. I don't know why you stay with me . . . I am unlovable."

*She Says:*

Premature forgiveness: "Well, since you will change, I guess I don't need to say the rest of how I feel."

### II. MOVING AWAY STYLE

*He Says:*

"I don't want to talk about it now."

*She Says:*

Not holding him accountable: "I know he wants to change, it's just hard for him."

### III. MOVING AGAINST STYLE

*He Says:*

"How dare you criticize me; I am the man here."

**Or**

"You're just like my mother, nag nag, nag . . ."

*She Says:*

Throw a life preserver: "Well, I didn't mean it like that; you really are a great guy. Let's just forget about what I said."

**Or**

Blame yourself: *"I am so sorry, I am really to blame . . ."*

**Or**

Emotional blackmail: *"If you love me, you will talk."*

**Or**

Being fragile: *"I will die if we don't talk right now!"*

**Or**

Tit for tat: *"Fine. I didn't really want to talk either, loser."*

**Or**

Emotional castration: *"Well, if you were a real man you would* [fill in the blank].

**Or**

Taking the momma bait: *"Well, I am nothing like your mother; I see I need to straighten you out about that first before I get back to what I was saying . . ."*

# Conclusion

Man defenses are born from individual histories, interpersonal skills, and personal dispositions. Taken together they form a predominant style of relating that under normal circumstances can be engaging and enjoyable. After all, you chose to be with this guy. However, under duress, a style slide can occur when an overdeveloped strength turns into a dysfunctional, rigid stance, disrupting the normal ebb and flow intimacy cycle. Each of us has points within the cycle that feel easy and others that are potentially sticking points, especially when we are not at our best. Understanding a person more fully can often lead to a more compassionate stance, even when they are being a pain. This ultimately makes giving feedback easier. This is a skill that needs to be mastered if relationships are to be successful with peers, partners, friends, or children.

# CHAPTER CUES

1. The man cam is an objective means to evaluate both strength and limitations, and to receive feedback.

2. The man cam develops when there is a history of people giving clear and accurate feedback. At some point, a man can be a source of credible feedback for himself.

3. The ebb and flow intimacy cycle suggests that moving toward, moving away, and moving against are all natural parts of any relationship. Most people have points in the cycle that they're comfortable with and others that need to be strengthened.

4. A disposition toward a specific point in the cycle eventually helps form a predominant style of relating and with it certain types of defenses:

   Skill $\longrightarrow$ Style $\longrightarrow$ Defense

5. Under duress, a style slide may occur when dispositional strengths turn into a potential liability in communication (defenses).

6. Knowing more about a man's personal history will often engender loving-kindness and understanding about man defenses.

7. Giving feedback in a systematic way can help avoid the many potential mishaps of the feedback process.

8. As a partner, family member, or friend, having a deeper understanding of your own personal history of the ebb and flow intimacy cycle, and where you may be prone to be derailed, will help in your efforts to communicate with your man.

# 11

## Why Every Man Needs a Guardian and How to Become One for the One You Love

Throughout this book, you have already gathered some tangible ways to help the men you love. In this chapter, we will take that to another level and discuss the central approach you can adopt to assist the males in your life: that of the "guardian." As we will see, being a guardian places you in a special type of relationship with a boy or man and allows you to help him. By taking this guardian stance, you will ultimately allow your son, husband, brother, or friend to discover or reorient himself toward his own unique version of being a man. The guardian helps accomplish this task through supplying special types of experiences that include support, challenge, providing information, clearing up conflicts, and helping heal past emotional wounds related to being a man. We have already looked at some of these skills earlier in the book when we learned about attunement, being a repackager for transforming difficult emotional situations, avoiding empathic failures, and recognizing V Spots.

This chapter will focus on combining some of these skills and adding new ones as well. While these individual skills can stand alone, cumulatively they result in the power to shape relationships in amazing ways. For instance, being a guardian for a young boy can help him discover a budding sense of individualism, and having these vital experiences in the formative years places his feet firmly on the path toward a healthy life.

Likewise, having a guardianlike relationship helps an adult (re)orient toward a deeper sense of authenticity, healing old wounds that otherwise haunt him and undermine many of his best efforts. The presence of a guardian can significantly impact his life, as well as the lives of his inner circle: romantic partner, family members, and friends. If a man has experienced the guidance of guardians in his life, he in turn has the potential to assume that same role for others. The care a guardian provides is vital, and its spirit is necessary in all stages of a male's life, from boyhood to old age.

It is important to point out right away that being a guardian involves a group of skills and a way of relating that almost everyone can learn. You don't have to be a trained mental health professional, nor is this approach limited by age or gender. Let's think of the guardian role as it compares to that of the male role model discussed in an earlier chapter. Remember the discussion about the male role model's gender-specific power to supply emotional support or guidance for boys or other men? The male role model provides a set of behaviors to imitate with no real consideration for developing a boy's own signature way of being a man. It comes in a one-size-fits-all approach. The male role model is also a gender-exclusive job: no females allowed. Because of other commandments involving fearing the feminine, women are often seen as a corrupting force in a male's quest for masculinity.

By contrast, the guardian approach is meant to be used in the real world by parents, peers, friends, and romantic partners—male and female alike. The only necessary requirement is the commitment to learn and implement the skills we discuss and fit them to your own style of relating. To understand more about the role of the guardian, we will devote a fair amount of time to describe the good care they provide.

The guardian is different from any other approaches found in today's self-help books for men in that it does not rest upon a foregone conclusion about how men should be ideally defined. The goal of most self-help books has been much like the old male-role-model version of masculinity: presenting a narrowly prescribed formula or checklist that is to be followed in order to become the ultimate man. Of course, this is often biased with the particular author's own beliefs and preferences related to political, spiritual, social, or religious values.

For the most part, these self-help approaches mean well, are usually evocative in their presentation, and emotionally moving for both men and women. People get high hopes that the secret lives of men have finally been discovered, and the one true way to be a man has been revealed. However, instead of creating lasting guidance for all men, what usually occurs is a serving up of the flavor of the month regarding manhood for a very select few. Those men for whom the latest manhood craze does not ring true are often left feeling even more bewildered and alienated from themselves and others.

Recently, I saw a morning talk show that highlighted the new fad for men this season, which apparently involves a return to some retooled version of stereotypical masculinity. This new ideal was presented as a less-manicured approach than the previous season's "metrosexual" or overly stylized heterosexual male. My first reaction upon hearing this was indignation—not that I had a lot of investment in the metrosexual fad, since most often I am found in a vintage pair of cowboy boots from the 1940s.

My irritation was more about the trendy ways that a core sense of individualism can be taken away and/or shifted by someone else's notion of fad masculinities. Much like last year's fashions, men are taught to shun who they are, or at least who they have been told to be, because it is out of step with the latest trend. This approach is fraught with problems, not because it tells men to adjust their clothing style with the times, but because it touches the accompanying deeper sense of "what's in" regarding their notion of being a man.

Tuning in each fall for the new line of manhood in order to keep in step with Madison Avenue separates men from their true sense of individualism and authenticity. Someone's true identity may be accentuated with minor ornamental updates but should not be subject to core retooling based on someone else's decision. Honoring the individual involves trusting that when the dust settles after hard-fought introspection and soul-searching, one cannot alter a man's core values without compromising his most essential nature. When this type of concession occurs, it weakens a man and his ability to function in the areas of work and love. Instead of drawing from core character that resonates in step with his own authentic being, he assumes the persona concocted by a whim or "authoritative" voice telling him to be someone he is not.

In terms of the logistics of living, life is demanding enough without the added burden of needing to deal with impression management in his most intense and intimate encounters. Losing who he is in the midst of a dual life, where he negotiates the tasks of work and love while keeping others away from his most private thoughts and feelings so they don't discover who he really is, can be burdensome. This is a built-in barrier to intimacy as well as a surefire way to drain his reservoir of energy in day-to-day functioning. The purpose of this chapter (and this entire book) is not to present a new fad with which men must conform, but rather to show men and their loved ones how to find or reconnect with their authentic selves. Being a guardian for a man you love can help him do this.

So how does the guardian help to defray and protect a man from these harmful influences? The guardian's job involves two main goals: (1) help those on the path to (re)discovering their core notion of manhood, and (2) honor, protect, and cultivate those authentic parts when they are revealed. As we will see, being a guardian is more than the warm, fuzzy moments that seem so effortless on Hallmark commercials. Instead, being a guardian is hard work, often pushing all those involved to personally stretch and grow.

One of the fundamental premises a guardian must understand is that there are a number of ways to be a healthy, happy man who is grounded in the ability to live peacefully in his own skin as well as make important and lasting connections with others. Not every healthy, happy man will look alike in these personal dimensions, nor should he. That is the power and splendor of the individual in the context of the larger society; we do not have to be carbon copies of each other to have good lives.

Instead of offering a simplified checklist of attitudes and behaviors to corral your man into accepting, we will do something more difficult and subsequently more lasting and beneficial. We will look at how a guardian sets up an environment that allows a male to discover who he really is, not what the latest trend tells him to be. Guardianship is experienced as a specific kind of relationship grounded in safety and care that in turn allows the authentic person to emerge from the persona, falsehood, and dysfunction that many males have experienced.

A guardian has the ability to determine the right balance of support and challenge needed in a man's life for him to grow. A man is encouraged to assume more mature responsibilities, and, when need be, heal old emotional wounds. He in turn picks up on the idea that it is okay to be himself. In this way, the guardian provides an unconditional sense of love, where the deepest part of a man remains protected by their care. A guardian also encourages him to continue down the road toward finding out who he really is as a man. I firmly believe these types of experiences, even when received well past the formative years, help a person in significant ways. It makes for a better life and allows emotionally arrested aspects in the heart and mind to suddenly find more emotional and psychological energy, and with it, more mature and responsible functioning.

While I use the term guardian throughout this chapter, it is important to note that its use has two potential applications: one with boys and one with men. Being a guardian for a boy versus a man differs on important dimensions like the balance of power in the relationship, the degree to which one person assumes responsibility for another, and even the degree to which certain emotional needs are supplied. Being a guardian for men can be thought of more along the lines of being an *ally* for them, emphasizing a more adult type of relationship. So, from here on, when "guardian" is mentioned, make the mental adjustment of who it is for, a boy or a man, and adjust for the appropriate level of expectations. As we will see, it is important to keep this guiding principle in mind.

# Meeting the Needs of Others:
# The Emotional Refueling Center

A guardian helps build and maintain the right environment in the relationship with some of the skills we have already discussed, like avoiding empathic failures and V Spots. It also involves the notion of supplying certain emotional needs. This can entail aspects like lending support, soothing hurt feelings, and giving encouragement in order to stretch in new ways. Experiences that fall under this category are meant to fill up a person emotionally, facilitating continued growth and healing

Imagine that everyone carries an internal reservoir for emotional needs and requirements. In growing up, the level to which it is filled often dictates one's eventual psychological health and functioning. There is a line on the gauge that indicates when enough needs have been met. When one crosses this line, there is a sense of having become a more whole and complete person; one has been changed in a permanent way. It affords new awareness and freedom about how one lives. Achieving this status is obtained through the steady care of at least one guardian, but it certainly helps to have more.

By contrast, when emotional needs go unmet on a chronic basis, the ill effects include not really knowing oneself or feeling thin-skinned and chained to past hurts. If requirements are not met in childhood, we still consciously and unconsciously seek to fill the emotional reservoir as adults. As we have seen, sometimes this occurs in both healthy and unhealthy ways.

One of the tasks of the guardian at times is to supply emotional needs for others, both boys and men. Psychoanalyst Margaret Mahler referred to the "emotional refueling center" that a caregiver provides for a child. That is, a caregiver fills up the emotional emptiness of the other person through the types of care and attunement we have discussed in this book. In a similar way, guardians can act as an emotional fueling center, where those who are in need often dock and feel the benefits of their care. When this notion is applied to boys, there is the implicit understanding that a parent acting as a guardian has a more comprehensive role as a nurturer. They will take greater responsibility for making sure the child's needs are met, as they are the central figure in supplying them. As the boy faces new challenges and dilemmas, some related to defining his budding notion of being a man, his resources may become temporarily tapped. Understandably, he will frequently need to take in nurturance from the guardian to refill his reservoir. However, having been filled enough times by the good care of a guardian, his inner world takes on a new shape and becomes more stable and solid. Though he is still subject to the slings and arrows of life, he bounces back more quickly and with less disruption.

This new steady status will also enable him to progressively assume a more active role in meeting his own needs (and eventually caring for others). So an integral part of the guardian's role is challenging the boy to grow in these more appropriately independent ways. For instance, in some shared moments, guardians sometimes have to encourage the child (or even young adult) to assume greater responsibility in what can be difficult moments of fledgling independence. He may feel uncertain of that next step in what is a long series of strides toward more mature functioning. These are crucial moments when the right balance of support and challenge are offered.

Other times he stretches on his own, because realistically speaking, the guardian cannot hover over the boy, adolescent, or young adult all the time. Sometimes parents really stress out when they imagine their child in these moments. They wonder: when confronted with life's challenges, will he make the right choices? In the best of situations, he draws upon the recollection of the guardian as an inspiration to find courage to go out into the world, meet new people, or even learn to manage for himself. He accomplishes another step toward a more mature, fulfilling life.

However, it is important to realize that even having successfully accomplished these new milestones, he will still occasionally come back "home" when overwhelmed or in need of special bolstering. Sometimes this is seen well into adulthood when he reconnects with his guardian through actual visits, phone calls, or e-mails. Other times, he reaches out to the memory of his guardian, one that has become a permanent part of his heart and mind. As a guardian, you have an extra-special opportunity to shape the core of his very being, becoming the voice that he hears when in distress or one that provides guidance in pivotal moments. This is the most powerful legacy you can leave your child. He literally carries you as a guardian for the rest of his life.

Given the backdrop of the Commandments, we cannot assume that all men have received this type of good care or had their emotional tanks filled enough to function with the type of independence required to carve out who they are as men. And even if they did, there is still the ongoing need for all human beings (men and women alike) to occasionally dock with their adult versions of the emotional refueling center. In the best adult relationships (partner or friend) there is definitely a supportive environment present, and having certain emotional needs met is a part of continued growth and, if need be, healing.

What is different about the guardian relationship regarding adult men is that there are adult expectations and responsibilities. For instance, a romantic partner acting as a guardian for a man should not assume she has adopted a new son per se, having to raise him, put up with tantrums or dangerous irresponsibility; nor should a guardian's role be construed as enabling "little boy" behavior and thereby conferring a permanent manchild status on an adult.

Care is given for many reasons, one of which is allowing even a wounded man to progressively assume a more mature and responsible stance in his life. In certain pivotal moments, this invitation to growth can seem as awkward as a wobbly legged boy taking his first steps toward maturity. This can also be especially taxing for the guardian, who is attempting to maintain the right balance of support and challenge, even in the face of often uncomfortable situations.

In cases where there is a difficult legacy of emotional wounds that needs to be dealt with, a guardian can be very helpful on a man's journey toward healing, but it is ultimately his responsibility to take those important steps. In these situations, the goal is that enough needs are being meet in a guardianlike way to help him move forward from his emotionally frozen past. The path to emotional health involves having a prerequisite level of needs satisfied. The old formula of males doing without, sucking it up, and moving on makes a boy or a man fragile and underdeveloped, leaving his inner tank empty. There is nothing there to draw upon in terms of caring for himself, much less anyone else in his life.

At the same time, the experience of guardianship is not a permission slip for men to stay emotionally arrested even when life has dealt them some difficult blows. Remember, the goal of being a guardian for both boys and men is to help them assume an active role in meeting their own needs while never losing sight that being in relationships is a central part of any healthy human being's functioning. This realization will allow them to shape how they wish to be as men. It helps them become more responsive and respectful partners, friends, and parents.

## ▶ Toolbox Tip: Growing Pains

As a therapist, I have come to deeply trust that the guardian's role of supplying the right balance of support and challenge is necessary for growth and healing. However, this does not mean that every time this blueprint is used, it is easily put into action. I still have moments when I see another struggling that take me off guard, usually endearing them to me and making me wish they could walk an easier path toward a more mature and responsible life. This often occurs when a painful past recollection is revealed for the first time and felt in a very deep way, or when a person confronts a present-day challenge that stretches them in ways beyond their comprehension (and comfort).

In these moments, the adult face before me is often replaced with the tender vulnerability and desperation of a little child, pleading to be released from the task at hand. "Do I have to? But it hurts to do that!" In these moments, there is sometimes the temptation to release the adult (and me as well) from what needs to be done. "It's okay" or "don't worry" are words that come to my mind. "We can come back to these issues another time," I seem to rationalize in my own head, even though I know this is the right moment to go forward with them. What often keeps me grounded in these instances is the realization that the person in front of me is quite literally experiencing growing pains, which are always uncomfortable and, in some circumstances, heartbreaking. But it is by passing through these moments and the accompanying tasks that an opportunity for a better life is created. The best response I often muster is, "I am sorry; I know it is hard, and I will walk through it with you as much as I can, while you do what needs to be done."

While there is a priority to maintain an ongoing relational environment of safety and trust, there are certain moments when the guardian takes on a more intense role. When the guardian is aware of and attuned to the needs of the other person, sometimes "bells go off," indicating there is a need to step up and provide a more special level of care. There are moments when guardians help create a psychological space that allows for self-exploration, extra empathy, and trust. While guardians are not responsible for providing the ultimate answers, they can assist a male through this process of discovering his own signature way of being a man. This can include acting as a sounding board when the pieces of his life seem to come apart in the face of frustration and confusion. In these moments, guardians turn up the volume and intensity as they look with kind, accepting eyes at the person before them. This might include aspects like being attuned to, and very aware of, what the person is saying and working hard to understand how it affects them. It can also involve special instances when damaged parts of his psyche and heart are revealed. Tending to these parts in the right way helps males get back on track, which in turn allows them to eventually become healthier and more fully functioning people.

If you are a parent, being a guardian will allow your boy to take steps toward manhood. If you're a spouse or friend, remember that giving this type of care to your significant other or friend allows some of those positive qualities to take root in his own psyche. In the long run, acting as a guardian represents an investment in helping to develop a more emotionally responsive partner or companion. This sets a standard in the relationship that is achievable and realistic, and it promotes reciprocity as well. In the end, he will be able to support you in the same fashion that you have supported him.

The type of care that a guardian supplies helps build a more content person (boy or adult). Living in such an authentic manner becomes the wellspring of creativity, peace, meaning, and grounding in life. A male's task (in all honesty, a part of everyone's journey) is ultimately to cultivate that type of existence. One of the key aspects of guardianship is empathic attunement, which is revisited in more detail in the next section.

## Empathic Attunement

In the last chapter, we looked at the painful legacy of empathic failures. Now we return as well to the opposite way of relating: empathic attunement. Your ability to utilize empathy will be the cornerstone of acting as a guardian. In extreme situations—when people feel upset, confused, or vulnerable—it is as if they go from their normal state of being, which is a cohesive whole, to becoming a collection of fragmented bits. It may seem like a giant mirror is suddenly breaking into shattered shards. In these moments, the person needs someone to respond to him in a way that will help bring the pieces back together. The job of a guardian at these times of crisis is to be in tune with what is needed in order for the person to feel better and sort things out. This is accomplished through listening to the other person in an empathic way.

Empathy, or the ability to be in tune with another's perspective, allows a guardian to be aware of the individual's inner world. In these cases, guardians are able to place themselves in the other person's shoes and understand at a deeper level what is troubling him. It is important for the guardian to understand and respond from the frame of reference of the other person. We can define empathic attunement as (1) being in harmony with what someone needs in various moments of vulnerability (remember this list of emotions includes those like hurt or frustrations and also joy and accomplishments), and then (2) responding in sync.

First, let's place this concept of being a guardian in a parent/child context as an example. When a parent can place himself or herself in the child's shoes and make appropriate responses, this makes the child feel understood and attended to, which automatically makes the situation easier to bear (for everyone!). This experience of trying to see from someone else's perspective reaches its extreme when dealing with a newborn and trying to figure out exactly what the infant wants when he is crying: "Is it gas? Is he hungry? Does he need a clean diaper?" The parent eventually begins to read the child's needs: "When he does this, there is a good chance it means this or that." Remember, even infants have a signature way of expressing these aspects, and it is the guardian's job to decipher what may initially seem like a secret code. But there is a big payoff emotionally and psychologically when taking the extra steps to do this: the child feels understood and, subsequently, it deepens the sense of trust and security in the relationship.

The importance of empathic attunement will find its way across the life span as well; for instance, as the boy grows up, you may have to field some vulnerable topics that are in need of a guardian's care. The mark of empathic attunement is being on the lookout for these occurrences and dealing with them as they arise. He may have questions about whether he is "being masculine" because he is not like all the other boys at school. He may have heard someone say, "A real man acts this way, but not that way," and he feels confused. Or maybe he tells you that he failed himself or someone important to him because he acted in a certain way. These are serious matters, ones that leave boys (and men also) in vulnerable, fragmented states.

When you are acting in the role of guardian for an adult man, the need for empathic attunement is likewise present. Being a guardian involves knowing an adult man's signature way of expressing his wants, needs, frustrations, and joys. As a partner or friend, knowing his rhyme and rhythm is equally important as you show your familiarity with the important landscape of his inner world. He may still have leftover issues from childhood that haunt him and could use a sounding board in moments when old emotional wounds feel tender and raw.

A prime time for this is around family visits, holidays, or anything that places him in contact with old hurts or messages about being a man that really didn't fit or were (and have continued to be) potentially damaging to him. Your role in these crucial moments is to be attuned to his emotional well-being and help take away some of the sting. But empathic attunement is not just limited to being attuned to vulnerable moments, making peace with the past, and shadow parent issues; it is also operative during his best moments, when you commemorate his authentic and healthy choices about being his own man.

## ▶ Toolbox Tip: Empathic Attunement in Moments of Crisis

In moments of confusion or temporary crisis, the best remedy is for the guardian to listen, try to understand, and then convey what the individual is feeling (remember to keep in check the common knee-jerk reaction to reference your own experiences or point of view if you were in the same situation at some point). That is, the guardian should reflect back to the person what he feels or simply acknowledge to him that his hurt is real. One of the most powerful and simple ways to do this is to say, "I am sorry. I know that hurts." After the emotions are soothed, sometimes advice may be given about how to handle the situation, and appropriate encouragement may occur. Mind you, these are not easy skills for everyone to acquire. They take time and patience to develop. Hopefully, as the relationship with your male (boy or man) grows, so does your understanding of his signature way of expressing pain or confusion. One of the most nurturing things in any type of relationship is having a predictable and reliable person in those moments.

# Seeing the Man You Love

The same spirit of empathy mentioned above is the basis for a guardian's ability to *see* when a male is genuinely being his own man. This entails noticing and honoring when people are authentically being themselves versus some assumed persona. Seeing someone is a multifaceted skill that for many people involves development and fine-tuning. It begins with the ability to recognize subtle nuances of personhood emerging and crescendos in the ability to celebrate a male being his own person.

A guardian learns to recognize authentic parts of his or her man shining through all the clutter connected to well-meaning but misdirected mandates from family, society, or himself. However, often the largest barrier, as we will see in the next section, involves a partner's, parent's, or friend's own biases regarding how they wish their man to be. They may see their man truly being himself, but it is just not the self they want to embrace. "Honey, would you mind being a little more like [fill in the blank]?" All of these conflicting messages and preconceptions stand in the way of really embracing his notion of who he is. However, for now let's tackle the task of just seeing and recognizing someone's authentic parts.

Since the earliest days of psychology, many have noted how our identity is built in the context of important others. What parents, partners, siblings, friends, and family notice, and subsequently label as "good" or "bad," goes a long way in determining if we ever show those parts of ourselves again or even allow them to further develop. In the best situations, there is a near-magical occurrence when a person of any age displays some part of his unique person and others respond in a guardianlike fashion. This begins in the early stages of self-exploration as a child.

For instance, a boy may watch how his parent responds when he shows his bent for adventure, sensitivity, intellectual curiosity, physical or emotional toughness, and so on for the first time. If the parent acknowledges this part of the boy (through gestures like a smile or a nod of the head, or words like "I like what you did . . ."), he feels emotionally validated. The child feels as if that revealed part of him is real and valuable. Also, when a caregiver *sees* him, it helps the child see himself. The boy begins to recognize and own more of the skills and talents that will shape his authentic notion of being a man. It also encourages him to continue developing this particular aspect of who he is as it gets labeled "good" or "worthy," both by the loved ones who gave it attention or admiration and, consequently, by himself.

This is how the authentic sense of being a person is slowly cultivated under the steady care of those who act as guardians for the fledgling parts of the self that have not quite come into their own, those that need the gentle encouragement and protection of others in order to be sustained. This process continues throughout childhood, as more of the unique sense of who he is develops. The bits and pieces coalesce over time to form a solid sense of who he is.

When someone feels the presence of a guardian, it helps self-identity blossom; likewise, the absence of such good care leaves certain parts to wither, or, as we have noted earlier in the book, it leads males to place vulnerable emotional parts into their "secret shoe box." Only in the security of solitude might some males allow that material to see the light of day. Or worse, those real parts of who he is get arrested, never becoming what they could have been under the proper care of a guardian.

The material of a male's inner world is tricky because, as a result of the Male Commandments, there is a simultaneous wish and fear to be known by others. Many boys and men really wish to be seen by those in their inner circle, while at the same time they fear a replay of past events when painful and derailing empathic failures occurred. However, whether one is under the sway of stringent societal demands or free to be his own man, all males still need to be seen by those they love. It feeds their inner world, helps with self-discovery and personal growth, and deepens relational connections. Acting with the spirit of a guardian can be a generative force for a male of any age. There is an innate psychological need to be seen and accepted for who we are by the significant others in our lives. This begins early in childhood and never goes away, from boyhood all the way to adulthood and old age.

Because a guardian cannot be everywhere at once, he or she needs to be on the lookout for the real person who is emerging in the midst of the pressures that can cause a male to stray from the true direction of his own internal compass. As many have noted in recent years, boys can especially experience a critical period of development when many issues can potentially shape the rest of their lives. Peer pressures, media messages about being a man, and wanting to please others can all make an impact, causing them to lose themselves in the process.

Though men have likely acquired more internal resources to buffer themselves by adulthood, they are not free from these pressures either. They can wish to appease those they love, such as a wife or friends, or feel the sway of coworkers, a boss, and so on, sometimes to their own detriment. Guardians can really help their man slowly shake off years of societal or familial expectations of what it means to be a man. They can also take this care a step further in tough moments by interceding before the full force of a situation is felt, acting as temporary shields and fending off incoming assaults. A guardian who has adjusted to the appropriate level of care can say things like, "You have not seemed like yourself lately; is something bothering you at school [or work, in that relationship, and so on]?" The result of this type of care, which shows that a guardian is paying attention, is that a male (boy or man) can feel safe enough to reveal who he is under the clutter. This is a powerful experience as they begin to hatch and break through the shell of falseness that may have imprisoned them.

Beyond recognizing an authentic part of the self is the next level of skill, and it is a powerful one. It involves celebrating the individual. A guardian's job in this area involves seeing the real person emerging and commemorating a man in moments of genuineness when his "man-o-meter" rings loud and true. This does not mean you give him a plaque or hand him a gift certificate for home electronics; the biggest reward is sincere appreciation, making him know that you are proud of him for being his own person.

This is like turning up the volume on your power to see him for all the small steps he has taken along the way, and saying things like, "I know you have been working really hard on [fill in the blank] the past six months, and I just want you to know how happy I am for you." Or, "I just want you to know that I am so glad you are my man" (or, son, or, friend). I guarantee there is no greater reward for a man than having his loved ones make these gestures. The power of this has an indescribable effect not only on deepening the intimacy of a relationship between two people but also on healing the wounds related to those who could or would not see the male for who he really is. When a person is in touch with those genuine aspects, life feels easier in the inner world.

Living more comfortably in his own skin also makes for a smoother flow in interactions with others. When this happens enough, a man learns to treasure these vital parts of his person and continues to hone them over time; they are what give a person his signature way of being a man. As the next Toolbox Tip reveals, a guardian also develops the ability to see when his or her man is engaged in the opposite of authenticity, when persona, cool poise, or mandates from others lead him to be someone he is not.

▶ **Toolbox Tip: Seeing What Does Not Fit**

Guardians in the form of a parent, partner, or friend will begin to notice characteristics that don't fit with a person's budding sense of masculinity. They make note of these things and gain confidence in the idea that they can read their boy or man's reactions. For instance, they see their child trying to please or put on a front, when in reality this way of behaving does not "click" for him in an authentic way. When this type of behavior occurs too often, the result is often stunted growth. A sense of falseness can potentially develop because the male is more concerned with his parents' (or others') wishes for him than searching for his own authentic path. Likewise, a grown man caught in the cycle of pleasing boss, romantic partner, or ghosts from his past is emotionally hobbling the real person from emerging. So being empathically attuned means not only seeing someone for who they are and what fits for them, but also seeing what does not fit. You come to understand what makes them tick.

# Keep Your Own "Man-tudes" in Check

You might remember as a little girl beginning to form snippets of your ideal man. They may have come from fictional characters in books, movies, or interactions with real people like your father or father figures. These also include experiences with friends, peers, and romantic interests from puppy love to your first kiss to the first time you really gave your heart to a man. You may have formed an ideal composite figure from experiences when a male was caring and sincere, declaring his love, or when you felt the most safe, wrapped in a man's arms, or when the most genuine aspects of yourself were seen and appreciated.

Building the template for the perfect man is also established through less joyful and tender moments like misunderstandings or rejections, such as when you sent that note to the cute boy in your junior high class that said, "I like you; do you like me? Check yes or no," and the answer was no. Experiences like horrible blind dates or long-term relationships that didn't work out can also help form your idea of the perfect partner.

All these situations were pivotal moments, both good and bad, when you made mental notes about what you liked, and equally important, what you did not. All these incidents began to create a picture of how your ideal man looks and acts. This image in your mind's eye is what we will refer to as your "man-tudes": the set of expectations, hopes, and dreams, including personality and physical attributes, that form your notion of a perfect man. Taken together, they may stir up feelings of longing, desire, safety, and love.

Now the hard part: holding the picture of the perfect man in your mind, then placing it beside your current boyfriend, spouse, or love interest. "Yikes! Hold on . . . what the hell happened!!!?" may be a common reaction to some of the discrepancies you suddenly see. If the man you fell for does not line up perfectly, some inconsistencies may be allowed. This may be especially true if a more hopeful, long-term trajectory can be seen.

I have certainly heard a number of people (both male and female) make reference to their future spouse as if they were a house on the real estate market awaiting inspection and appraisal: "Yes, they are a real fixer-upper, but all the basics are there," or, "They just need a little touch-up work." However, if over the course of the relationship some of those new additions that were hoped for never took shape, or worse, the grand remodeling in no way occurred, there may be a sense of feeling a little cheated.

Some part of you may believe if your partner or husband were more like your ideal man, everyone would be happier, right? This wish for him to change could be based on an inventory of your own hurts that need mending or desires going unfulfilled. You believe your partner's metamorphosis would set those things right. Of course, a little rationalization can help you convince yourself that he would also benefit from the transformation. If you are in a committed relationship, you may feel left with the potential dilemma: do you try to change the man you have into the man you've always wanted?

The remainder of this discussion will focus on when changing is healthy for him, and to what degree. Knowing the difference between your man's natural dispositions versus areas where he could use some fine-tuning is helpful. A man's authentic self is based on his own individual hardwiring. Not all men are the same, and variability along personality dimensions/ traits is expected across a wide population. For instance, some men are natural thrill seekers, others even-keeled; some are gregarious, others introverted.

We could make an exhaustive list of dispositional qualities, some of which are the core elements for your man's individual identity. That core part of who he is at the foundation affects, among other things, his notion of being a man. Disavowing those aspects means compromising the fundamental nature of who he is at the center of his being. The spirit of this book endorses the premise that men become healthier and happier when they are assisted in developing and embracing their true nature, not deviating from it. Asking a man to deny who he is imposes a double whammy of unrealistic and unhealthy expectations. Attempts to take on that type of Herculean task result in an imposter cozying up next to you in bed, not the real person you chose.

Now, there are two other matters that need to be explained, which we will refer to as (1) "tightening up the authentic self" and (2) working on the underdeveloped side of the personality through personal growth, or working on the "masculine shadow." While you do a man a deep disservice by asking him to be someone he is not, you are well within bounds when asking him to tighten up his act, even when it lines up with his authentic self. Just because a man is in touch with his true disposition does not mean that it is all squared away and fully functioning at his highest level.

One of the best TV shows that illustrates the spirit of tightening up the true self is *Queer Eye for the Straight Guy*. I like this show because the consultants who give a man-makeover do not ask a man to change the fundamental nature of who he is; instead, they just suggest that he do it better. So, if their client has a thing for "sports attire," suggestions are made about showing that part of himself in other ways besides wearing dirty, holey sweatpants from the 1980s. This approach may also include trying something new that still reflects his signature approach, like a new haircut, clothing, and grooming habits. Again, this is all done within the bounds of the man's own personality style. They also pick up on areas that need fine-tuning regarding the interpersonal arena, like expressing themselves to their partners; they don't ask them to go outside of their own personal mode of operation, they just help them improve it.

We should also take the tightening-up notion one step further by making a distinction between genuinely healthy and genuinely unhealthy aspects of the masculine self. Lots of self-help jargon will direct people to be "genuine," the spirit of which seems very nice and uplifting. The problem is that some people's genuine self in its present state is not healthy. Case in point: when you have a man who is addicted to online gambling and will not face the deeper pain that drives his addictive behavior. He complains angrily that his partner's pleas for him to get help infringe upon his genuine self; after all, he is just embracing his authentic nature, which loves the thrill that accompanies risk taking.

Or what about a man who is so reserved that he enjoys the richness of his inner world but fails to include important others (including you) in it? Those who embrace the type of logic that authenticity implies a perfect state of being, even if it is harmful to himself or others, miss the point by employing it as an excuse for continuing destructive behaviors that are authentic but unhealthy. Often these misconceptions are the result of the Ten Commandments of Growing Up Male and other failed societal/ familial mandates or personal misfires that hurt everyone.

The authentic self is not necessarily pristine, and at times it can reveal primal aspects that need to be tamed, mended, or healed. This is especially true if there is a legacy of the Commandments hanging over a man's head. For many men, their true self is more like an unfinished painting—the initial lines are there but the residue of the past keeps the final canvas from being filled in. Helping someone discover his genuine disposition may reveal areas that are raw, sharp, and cause your man pain. While all of these are authentic parts of him, they are not authentically healthy. Becoming more authentic in these areas of the psyche and heart involves making peace with the past, changing behavior, and becoming a better parent, partner, or friend. Sometimes this means going to therapy to gets things squared away.

Beyond helping a man find his true disposition and mend his broken parts, there is also the potential for another type of experience related to personal growth. There are a number of theories in psychology that talk about becoming a more fully functioning, whole, or individuated person. Carl Jung suggested that the mission of the first half of life was finding our true dominant personality style; this is very much akin to the discussions at various points in this book about learning to be one's own man. After these are in place, we direct most of our lives with our innate strengths leading the way. For the most part, that is a very good thing, but sometimes a problem can develop when well-worn approaches turn into overdeveloped strengths, making the personality a bit lopsided. For instance, a person who has worked hard most of his life developing his powerful, in-control stance may leave other aspects like tenderness or vulnerability behind. Likewise, a creative, sensitive type may hone those qualities to the exclusion of more dependable or sturdy traits, affecting his efforts in work and love.

At some point (usually around midlife, though more contemporary analysts believe this process can happen earlier), Jung believed an unbalanced feeling would begin to make itself visible on a person's radar screen, alerting the individual that something is missing. It may also be brought to one's attention by others who convey, in both direct and indirect ways, that an overdeveloped strength is causing some friction. An overdeveloped quality can dominate the whole personality, not leaving room for the creation of other new avenues of healthy relating and living.

Jung suggested that the task of the second half of life, then, was adding balance by working on areas that were underdeveloped. Underdeveloped areas are by definition ones that have stayed dormant, lag behind, or feel like they cut against the grain. Jung referred to these aspects as our "shadow" side. For some, that may conjure up sinister images of split personalities like Dr. Jekyll and Mr. Hyde, but what it really refers to is the stunted part of us that remains in the shadow of our more dominant side for most of our lives. Like a tree in the woods that does not receive its share of sunlight, it does not have the opportunity to grow.

Jung argued that the goal of becoming a fully functioning person is realized by bringing the shadow aspects of our personality into the light and then doing the necessary work to cultivate them. This allows a person to become more whole and fully integrated, incorporating all of his parts and marshaling his complete forces. The man who has spent most of his life learning to be powerful and in control learns about the joy of surrender; the man who has spent his life enriching his emotional life can come to know the sense of bridling and directing his feelings in a purposeful way. Doing this shadow work is about filling in the other side of the equation. It is more than just fine-tuning an already existing area; it involves adding something new to the picture. Often it involves the mirror opposite of the core dominant side of the personality.

Now we need to take this concept of working on the underdeveloped side of the personality and apply it directly to masculinity. We will refer to this as the "masculine shadow," or the underdeveloped or opposite of a man's dominant disposition. On pages 334–335 is a list of dominant qualities that may pop into your mind as you think of your man's signature style of relating. Accompanying these more dominant traits are the likely underdeveloped aspects that wait to be cultivated.

A man's goal in this next step of growth is to begin bringing these personality aspects into being as a necessary step toward a more whole life. One of my favorite people from my training as a psychologist was the director of the counseling center where I did my internship. Besides being a genuinely nice person, he seemed very comfortable in the role of all of the meet-and-greet activities that accompanied his position at the center. He appeared gregarious, comfortable in his own skin, and able to draw others into conversation whether willing or not, like some pied piper of the psychological realm.

This all seemed to come so easily for him. I found out differently one day as we had coffee. He told me that the social part of his job was at one time the most tasking. I discovered he was by nature fairly reserved, and while he enjoyed being with people, he had to push himself into learning about being more outgoing. While the end results obviously served him well, he had come to appreciate and even enjoy his new skill set, but it really was hard work getting there.

In the process of developing his shadow side he was aware that "being on" would sometimes leave him drained, in need of alone time to recharge his batteries and think through fine-tuning his new skills. Working on that underdeveloped side was a back-and-forth process, and as true for most of us, it involved the occasional fall on his face. The point may be obvious, but this masculine shadow work is hard!

What accompanies this process is often anxiety about not being enough. What we also need to keep in mind is that the masculine shadow side has other emotional qualities associated with it, like embarrassment (e.g., "I wish people didn't know that about me"), or awkwardness ("I don't like feeling incompetent"), or for some, downright shame ("People used to make fun of me because of this . . ."). For all of these reasons, underdeveloped areas are not high on many people's to-do list. Instead, people shy away from them, or worse, bury them deep out of sight.

For some men, these negative associations with their shadow sides are further enhanced because of the weight of the Commandments and their messages about needing to be powerful and proficient at every task undertaken. This sets up what feels like a Darwinian "survival of the fittest" that does not allow for men to realize moments of vulnerability or inhabit the student role that often accompanies work in the shadow realm. Research supports one of the difficulties with men going to therapy; they assume that being in such a circumstance means another humiliating chapter from their man-training experience. And then, of course, men sometimes do not do this masculine shadow work because of another added wrinkle regarding rigid relationship patterns.

## ▶ Toolbox Tip: Masculine Shadow

Below you will find a general but certainly not exhaustive list of core-developed dispositions and the opposites that often accompany them. Use this list as a starting point for a man's shadow work. Remember, this list can be read in either direction, where some shadow side traits are actually men's dominant dispositions and vice versa.

| DOMINANT SIDE | MASCULINE SHADOW SIDE |
| --- | --- |
| Rational | Feeling |
| Meticulous | Intuitive |
| Creative | Steady |

| Dominant Side | Masculine Shadow Side |
|---|---|
| Spontaneous | Creature of habit |
| Adventurous | Safe |
| Stoic | Emotionally accessible |
| Gregarious | Contemplative |
| Sexually primal | Emotionally tender |

One of the more complicated issues addressed in this book is the masculine shadow and its impact on the romantic connection. As his partner, you may have chosen him (consciously or unconsciously) based on shared values and interests but also because of the ways he complements your strengths and weakness. That is a nice way of saying you and he may be mirror opposites in some significant ways. In many couples there is an unspoken and often unaware contract regarding the allocation of important duties and responsibilities.

When two people come together, the relationship begins to represent the merger of two people's histories, families, and financial resources, but also things like life skills and deficits. It is as if you begin to form your own company with you and your partner as owners and operators. There are certain areas in the corporation that are run exclusively by one person, whereas others are shared in various degrees. There is the travel agency, which supplies directions, the front office where executive decisions are made, the child-care area, the romance department, and telecommunications regarding friends, family, and so on. These roles are firmly established, creating specific relationship patterns. This extends beyond who will be in charge of the finances, disciplining the kids, or doing the laundry. It often involves who carries certain emotional responsibilities like power, control, emotions, rational decision making, adventure, sexuality, stability, and so on in the relationship.

Couples get entrenched in their rhythm of how things are done; this can go on in both functional and dysfunctional ways over the course of a lifetime. Both people may feel locked into their jobs and duties because deviations from roles cause anxiety in the relationship. Rest assured, the deviant spouse is often quickly ushered back into his or her familiar responsibility, even if the change could potentially mean a good payoff in the long run. Sometimes, when these entrenched roles cause too much conflict, a marital therapist may need to be consulted to help break the couple's dysfunctional patterns, as well as to help manage the attendant worry and anxiety that arises in such an exercise.

Fixed relationship patterns can provide predictability over the years, but they can also potentially impact the man's ability to do masculine shadow work; in addition, it can impact a woman's capacity of performing her own shadow work. Earlier in the book, we discussed a common relationship agreement where the man provides stability, acting as the day-to-day emotional rock in moments of upset (a common stereotypical male role). When this relationship pattern is too rigid, it may lead to lopsidedness in his ability to be more fully functional. This hones his dominant skill set but leaves other abilities, like awareness of his own emotional state, far out of reach, tucked away in the shadowy recesses of his mind. Many partners' justified complaints about wishing he could/would do [fill in the blank] better are rooted in their man's ability to transcend old roles. When one partner begins to break the relationship rules through choice or circumstances (e.g., going back to school, having a baby, physical illness, etc.), it opens the window to potential change for both partners to have a fuller life.

Some may wonder, "Is this masculine shadow work really necessary? What would happen if he opts out of this part?" As with most answers provided in this book, there are few sweeping generalizations and a number of individual scenarios. There will be a range of men whose sense of masculinity stays overshadowed in various degrees by their dominant side. For some men, that may not throw things off-kilter in a way that significantly harms his functioning; he just misses out on gaining that potential extra gear that could boost his level of success and happiness in work and love. Other men will be more drastically impacted to where the degree of lopsidedness often causes the man to be consistently off balance. Those men can be candidates for running through a series of relationships and jobs, alienating parents, partners, and friends. For these men, engaging the masculine shadow is a necessity.

Being committed to finding the buried treasure in the underdeveloped aspects of our identities can pay off in big dividends. Jung himself argued that the shadow side of a personality is predominately golden. The same can be said of his masculine shadow, as its development has direct implications for him and for you as his partner, friend, and so on. Helping a man step into his genuine sense of being is something that will pay off in the long run. He will be freer to be himself, and that means he will be able to relate to you in a more genuine way. This cuts across all areas: love, sex, and companionship.

We've circled back to where we started in discussing your man-tudes. As a partner, you may have always wanted a little something extra from your man, like a greater ability to share parts of himself, being able to stand on his own feet more firmly, or being in touch with the more creative or ambitious part of who he is. When these hopes are closer to the heart of your man-tudes, no doubt missing out on them will be more distressing at the individual level and within the relationship.

A legitimate request that can be beneficial for both of you involves encouraging your man to do his shadow work. This may up the odds that some of these hoped-for personality traits will become more developed. It also ushers in the possibility that, as his partner, you'll begin to realize underdeveloped areas as well. Couples, friends, and family all benefit from a man doing his shadow work.

## RELATIONSHIP RED ZONE:
### Building Your Perfect Man

Remember playing with paper dolls when you were a little girl? We are going to do a version of that now, but instead of trying to make Barbie's friend Ken, take a few moments to think about your ideal man. Imagine a cutout man and dress him up with the ideal characteristics on your man-tude list. Fill in words that describe these characteristics.

Next, imagine a second cutout man and write down those areas that don't match with the man you love. You shouldn't feel guilty or embarrassed about this, but you might not want to leave it in a picture frame near your bed either. Ask yourself, "What are the areas where I feel most pressured to make my husband or partner be like my ideal man?" The answer to that will be a Relationship Red Zone that may not only affect your biases but may inadvertently empathically fail the man you love. These need to serve as markers for where the danger zones may exist.

## ▶ Toolbox Tip: Trajectory of Personal Growth

Here is a summary for the trajectory of personal growth that a guardian can help with:

1. Discovering his true self
2. Helping the authentically damaged parts heal
3. Developing the underdeveloped side of his personality (masculine shadow work)

## ▶ Toolbox Tip: Guardians Are Involved with These Empathy Tasks

1. Being empathically attuned in moments of crisis (when acting as a repackager)

2. Being empathically attuned by seeing the man you love
3. Being empathically attuned by celebrating his notion of being a man
4. Being empathically attuned by keeping your own man-tudes in check
5. Being empathically attuned by creating a relationship atmosphere that helps a man discover or reorient himself to his genuine notion of being a man

# Various Kinds of Guardians Across the Life Span

Remember, a guardian can be found in many different types of relationships, including between a parent and child, amid friends, and certainly among significant others. Relationships geared toward man-making have, until now, been exclusively reserved in theory for the father or father figure, as reflected in the Commandments. However, the guardian approach is very different because we are not bound by old-fashioned gender constrictions; instead, men and women can both be guardians. Repackaging the complexity of life events in whatever shape, form, or time period is best done by those who act with the spirit of guardianship. Remember, having need of a guardian does not make him less of a man; it just reaffirms that he is human. To continue developing our understanding of the guardian role and how it works, let's look at a film example.

In the British movie *About a Boy*, Will (played by Hugh Grant), is a thirty-something womanizer who, through a series of interconnected events, meets a young teenage boy named Marcus. They become unlikely friends. Will is the epitome of cool; he knows the right clothes, music, and attitudes that impress others. That is, until they see beyond his shallow presentation. The boy, by contrast, is socially inept, has no friends, dresses in dated clothing, and gets bullied. The thing is, Marcus really has a sensitive, thoughtful side that is genuine and engaging. People who get to know him really like him. He just doesn't know how to get to that point very often.

Over the course of what seems like a mismatched friendship, Will and Marcus begin to rub off on each other in positive ways. Will learns more about finding the genuine parts of himself, and Marcus learns to be more socially poised. However, the boy's social gains are placed in jeopardy when it is discovered that he will sing a dated Roberta Flack song, "Killing Me Softly (with His Song)," at the school talent show. Making things worse, Marcus dedicates his performance to his depressed mother, who only finds joy in hearing her son sing. Will finds out about the concert at the last moment and rushes to the auditorium to dissuade Marcus, telling him, "This is social suicide." But Marcus feels this is still the right thing to do. As predicted, Marcus goes onstage, is roundly booed, and then freezes up. Before he leaves the stage, totally humiliated, Will grabs an electric guitar and accompanies Marcus as he sings. It suddenly turns into an event. Others seem surprised, yet are drawn to them.

In this situation, Will acted as a guardian for Marcus. He challenged Marcus's decisions socially about his identity as a man, but in this pivotal moment, he also realized that Marcus had to stick to his guns, even if it was something he wouldn't do in a million years. This is important, because men have their own man-tudes for themselves (and others), and the hope is they can keep them in check for their sons, friends, and family. Will's guardianship comes into full force as he supports Marcus, allowing him to be his own man but helping him fine-tune a bit.

You may also notice in this story that Will learns a thing or two from Marcus about being a more genuine man. In some ways, Marcus is a guardian for him. Marcus constantly challenges him on this front, encouraging Will to become more forthright with his romantic interest, the only woman with whom Will has ever had a semimature relationship. Will hesitates about this, believing his girlfriend would not like who he *really* is. In a critical moment, Marcus does agree that Will is "a bit blank" on the personality front, but the care he has experienced from him is genuine, and that is something that can be built upon. Will's days as a notorious womanizer draw to a close as he is finally able to develop and share more of who he is with others.

In this story, an unlikely pair become guardians for each other in various degrees. We see that part of acting in the spirit of guardianship is recognizing the genuine parts of the other person as he begins to define who he is as a man, but a guardian also challenges the other person to build upon the parts of himself that are authentic but in need of fine-tuning. In the movie, Marcus becomes more socially poised and comfortable within his own skin, and Will becomes more genuine in his relationships with others. Certainly, the sprit of this same kind of connection can be found between two adult men or two adolescent boys who are guardians for each other. Remember also that we are not bound by gender; the spirit of guardianship can involve a single mom who advocates on behalf of her son, a sister who provides care for a brother, or a wife who provides this type of care for her husband.

A good movie example of a woman acting as a guardian for a boy is *Billy Elliot*. In this film, a young working-class boy unexpectedly discovers he has a gift for dance, though his father would much rather he take up boxing. Billy's dance instructor both supports and challenges him as she deals with his frustration, anger, and confusion about being a dancer. He is very distressed that what seems so natural to him can be labeled as "wrong" by those close to him. It is through his dance instructor's steady guardianship that he eventually embraces his authentic nature.

There is a pivotal scene when Billy's father finally sees him dance and is won over, not only because he is so good but because it fits the boy so well. In this case, the guardianship becomes contagious, and other family members support Billy in embracing his authentic masculine self. This in turn not only deepens the father/son connection, but eases other family tensions as well. When one person takes on the mantle of guardian, usually everyone benefits in some way, and the effects are not limited to parent/child relations. As mentioned earlier, the hope in more adult relationships between friends or romantic partners is that guardianship is reciprocal. Ideally, in those cases, guardianship has a more give-and-take feel to it, with each person watching out for the other.

As mentioned earlier in the chapter, being a guardian is not easy work. It is more than just warm, touchy-feely experiences. Sometimes a guardian needs to be strong—for both people involved. Honest but caring challenges are made. Guardians have to stretch their protection over the other person, shielding them from external threats, such as those from society or from his family, who may tell him just how he should act to be considered a man. At other times, the biggest threats come from within, where damaging messages stemming from the legacy of the Commandments still echo in his heart and mind.

## ▶ Toolbox Tip: Barriers Across the Life Span

Below is a short list of barriers a man may encounter across his lifetime. They are potential places where challenges to one's notion of being a man may occur. Many of these are overcome more easily with the assistance of a guardian.

### Little Boy Barriers
- Earliest discovery of his sense of being a man
- Trying on different roles and personas to figure out what fits

### Young Man Barriers
- Committed romantic relationships
- Entering the world of work
- Learning about sex
- Neverland barrier

### Adult Barriers
- Negotiating being a grown-up in romantic relationships
- Having children—they become more important than your needs
- Gainful employment and success

### Midlife Barriers
- The body begins to slow down or not work as well
- Children may leave the nest
- Realizing that youthful fantasies may not come true
- Changes in long-term romantic relationships

- Changes in the nature of relationship with parents (them aging/becoming more dependent)
- Loss of parents

## Retirement and Aging Barriers

- The body breakdown
- Questioning your life's meaning
- Contemplating your own demise
- Contemplating your significant other's death
- More reliant on others for care

Finally, with the newfound freedom that the presence of the guardian brings, the Toolbox Tip below presents the "Counter Commandments," or answers to the cumbersome and restricting social norms men sometimes experience and which we have been looking at throughout this book. The original Commandment is presented first, followed by each Counter Commandment. These Counter Commandments reflect the spirit of healthy individualism that is obtainable when a man truly is his own man.

## ▶ Toolbox Tip: The Counter Commandments

| OLD COMMANDMENT | COUNTER COMMANDMENT |
|---|---|
| 1. There is only one way to be a man. | 1. There are a number of healthy ways to be a man. |
| 2. Fear the feminine. | 2. Men can learn that those aspects labeled as feminine are actually an innate part of all members of the human race. |
| 3. Men must funnel all their feelings into sex or aggression. | 3. Men can become competent and skilled in the use of all emotions. |
| 4. Affections is always associated with sex. | 4. Tender feelings do not always mean sexual feelings. |

| OLD COMMANDMENT | COUNTER COMMANDMENT |
|---|---|
| 5. You big ape: masculinity is based on power, strength, and paranoia. | 5. Men can discover their masculine shadow side and develop all aspects of their personality. |
| 6. A boy needs a male role model for his sense of being a man. | 6. A boy needs a guardian to realize his ultimate sense of being a man is flawed. |
| 7. If your father is rejecting, you must learn to please him. | 7. Finding peace with your shadow parent(s) allows for peace and more choice in your life as a man. |
| 8. If you don't please your mother, you must marry someone like her. | 8. Finding peace with your shadow parent(s) allows you to make better choices about romantic partners |
| 9. Being a man is a 24/7 job. | 9. A man's sense of masculinity is found in every avenue of his life and can serve as a vast resource, not a detriment. |
| 10. A man must follow the commandments even if it causes him to be emotionally stunted or leads him off track. | 10. The power of being your own man is carving out an authentic sense of individualism amid the inevitable pressures to conform to personas and other societal falsehoods. |

# Conclusion

In this chapter, we looked at how you can really help the males you love by assuming the role of guardian. The qualities displayed by a guardian help boys and men become their own men. Let's quickly review how a guardian can help raise boys. In the best situations, the basic building blocks for this process are established in the formative years. It is crucially important when guardians see and celebrate their son's individual, healthy sense of uniqueness, while keeping man-tudes in check. Caregivers who can act as guardians create an emotional/psychological environment that helps their son become his own man. This is at the heart of being a guardian. The good care that is provided, empathic attunement as well as the right balance of support and challenge, will eventually lead to the boy's developing his own sense of masculinity and enable him to decide how he wants to be as a man.

Just as a boy has not completed the process of becoming a man in the first few years of life, neither is the caregivers' job complete when they are assuming the role of the guardian. They may be asked to respond to the boy, then teenager, then young adult, then adult about his masculine concerns. Of course, although acting in a similar spirit to what was done in the formative years, the caregiver will be a different type of guardian at various stages of the male's development. The son may need different things at various points in his growth. The hand-holding as a child may give way to a more mature type of support as he gets older. The son at some point may even want a more adult relationship with his caregivers. He may ask real questions such as, "What was it like to be a man in your day; how did you deal with these types of troubles?" However, underneath these differing types of experiences lies the spirit of the guardian—the belief in the genuine sense of masculinity that his or her son adopts. With this belief comes the knowledge that this authentic spirit of masculinity will lead to a better life for him and those around him.

The point needs to be made that if you are going to act as a guardian for your son, it is crucial to get to know him, his interests, likes, and dislikes.

Over time, you get a feel for when your son is on track and when he is not. The guiding idea behind assuming the guardian role is that one should be able to discern when issues related to being a man need to be addressed. And don't assume this is a onetime discussion. A guardian may have to address this issue again and again. These discussions need to continue until that missing piece fits into place. At each stage, there comes a deeper and more complex notion for the boy and his growing sense of being a man. New subtleties surrounding this very complex issue of being a man arise. In addition, old issues may have to be recategorized or understood in a deeper way. Five-year-old boys have different notions of what it means to be a man than ten-year-olds, teenagers, or adults—but some of the same questions may be asked in different ways at differing stages of development.

It must also be remembered that many of today's men did not receive the type of good care described in this chapter. I believe that one reason for the continuing development of the recent men's movement is that adult men realize they missed out, and now they are trying to do something about it. In addition, there is a recognition that men fine-tune their notion of being a man throughout their lives as they encounter life's challenges and triumphs. In other words, a boy doesn't learn everything he needs to know about being a man while he's in kindergarten or the sandbox. In the normal course of life, sometimes even the sturdiest man is called upon to adapt to circumstances over which he has no control.

# CHAPTER CUES

1. A guardian is someone (male or female) who acts in your best interest, promoting an authentic, healthy sense of self.

2. Creating a spirit of guardianship involves establishing the right balance of support and challenge in a relationship.

3. In moments of crisis, a guardian turns up the volume on the relational environment, making it particularly safe for self-exploration and healing.

4. When acting as a guardian for a man, it is more in the spirit of an ally, maintaining the relational environment but also keeping adult expectations and responsibilities.

5. When acting as a guardian for a boy, the role of nurturer is more intense.

6. Empathy, or being attuned to another, is the core concept upon which the skills of being a guardian are based. This includes being empathically attuned in moments of crisis as well as recognizing authentic parts in others.

7. Man-tudes represent your list of ideal attributes for your man. It is important to realize them and keep them in check. Not doing so can result in an empathic failure.

8. A man's authentic self may be in need of fine-tuning, or under-developed aspects of his personality may need to be built up by doing masculine shadow work.

9. When a man does his shadow work, it often creates a psychological space in a romantic relationship that frees up old fixed roles. This can usher in a new period of growth for both partners.

10. A guardian is often needed across the life span as men encounter many potential challenges to their notions of what it means to be a man.

# REFERENCES

Addis, M.E. & Mahalik, J.R. (2003). Men, masculinity, and the contexts of help seeking. *American Psychologist*, 58 (1), 5–14.

Archer, J. & Cote, Sylvana. (2005). Sex differences in aggressive behavior: A developmental and evolutionary perspective. In R.E. Tremblay, W.W. Hartup & J. Archer (eds.), *Developmental Origins of Aggression* (425–446). New York: Guilford Press.

Bem, S.L. (1974). The measurement of psychological androgyny. *Journal of Consulting and Clinical Psychology*, 42, 155–162.

Blazina, C., Cordova, M., Pisecco, S., Settle, A.G. (2007). Gender Role Conflict Scale for Adolescents: Correlates with masculinity ideology. *Thymos, The Journal of Boyhood Studies*, 1, 191–204.

Blazina, C., Eddins, R., Burridge, A., & Settle, A. (2007). The relationship between masculine ideology, loneliness, and separation-individuation difficulties. *Journal of Men's Studies*, 15, 101–110.

Blazina, C. & Marks, L. (2001). Therapeutic treatment references for gender role conflicted men: The choice of psycho-educational groups, individual therapy, or men's groups. *Psychotherapy: Theory, Research, Practice, Training*, 38, 201–212.

Blazina, C., Pisecco, S., & O'Neil, J. (2005). An adaptation of the Gender Role Conflict Scale for Adolescents: Psychometric issues and correlates with distress. *Psychology of Men and Masculinity*, 6, 39–45.

Blazina, C., Settle, A., & Eddins, R. (2008). Gender role conflict and separation-individuation difficulties: Their impact on college men's loneliness. *Journal of Men's Studies, 16*, 70–82.

Blazina, C. & Watkins, C.E. (1996). Masculine gender role conflict: Effects on men's psychological well-being, chemical substance usage, and attitudes toward help-seeking. *Journal of Counseling Psychology, 43*(4), 461–465.

Blazina, C. & Watkins, C.E. (2000). Separation/individuation, parental attachment, and male gender role conflict: Attitudes toward the feminine and the fragile masculine self. *Psychology of Men and Masculinity, 1*, 126–132.

Blazina, C. (1997). The fear of the feminine in the western psyche and the masculine task of disidentification: Their effect on the development of masculine gender role conflict. *Journal of Men's Studies, 6*, 55–68.

Blazina, C. (1997). Mythos and men: Toward new paradigms of masculinity. *The Journal of Men's Studies, 5*, 193–202.

Blazina, C. (2001a). Analytic psychology and gender role conflict: The development of the fragile masculine self. *Psychotherapy: Theory, Research, Practice, Training, 38*, 50–59.

Blazina, C. (2001b). Gender-role-conflicted men's poor parental attachment and separation/individuation difficulties: Knights without armor in a savage land. *Journal of Men's Studies, 9*(2), 257–265.

Blazina, C. (2001c). Part objects, infantile fantasies, and intrapsychic boundaries: An object relation's perspective on male difficulties with intimacy. *The Journal of Men's Studies, 10*, 89–98.

Blazina, C. (2003). *The cultural myth of masculinity.* Westport, CT: Praeger.

Blazina, C. (2004). Gender role conflict and the disidentification process: Two case studies on fragile masculine self. *Journal of Men's Studies, 12*(2), 151–161.

Bowlby, J. (1969). Disruption of affectional bonds and its effects on behavior. *Canada's Mental Health Supplement, 59*, 12.

Bowlby, J. (1980). *Attachment and Loss.* New York: Basic Books.

Burke, R.J. (2000). Effects of sex, parental status, and spouse work involvement in dual career couples. *Psychological Reports, 87*(3), 919–927.

Clatterbaugh, K. (1998). *Contemporary Perspectives on Masculinity: Men, Women, and Politics in Modern Society.* Boulder, CO: Westview Press.

Connell, R.W. (1995). *Masculinities.* Berkeley: University of California Press.

Crick, N.R. & Grotpeter, J.K. (1995). Relational aggression, gender, and social-psychological adjustment. *Child Development, 66*, 710–722.

Darwin, C. (1872/2005). *The Expression of the Emotions of Man and Animals*. New York: Adamant Media Corporation.

Draghi-Lorenz, R., Reddy, V., & Costall, A. (2001). Rethinking the development of "non-basic" emotions: A critical review of existing theories. *Developmental Review*, 21, 263–304.

Fairbairn, W.R.D. (1952). *An Object Relations Theory of Personality*. New York: Basic Books.

Fischer, A.R. & Good, G.E. (1997). Men and psychotherapy: An investigation of alexithymia, intimacy, and masculine gender roles. *Psychotherapy*, 34, 160–170.

Franz, M.L. Van. (1970). *Puer Aeternus: A psychological study of the adult struggling with the paradise of childhood*. New York: Sigo.

Freud, S. (1905). *Three Essays on the Theory of Sexuality* (Vol. 7). London: Hogarth Press.

Freud, S. (1963). Observations on wild psychoanalysis. In P. Rieff (ed.), *Freud: Therapy and technique*, 89–96. New York: Macmillan.

Freud, S. (1920). *Beyond the Pleasure Principle. Standard Edition of the Complete Works of Sigmund Freud*, 18, 3–64.

Freud, S. (1937). *Analysis Terminable and Interminable. Standard Edition of the Complete Works of Sigmund Freud*, 23, 209–253.

Gilligan, C. (1982). *In a Different Voice*. Cambridge: Harvard Press.

Gennep, A. Van, (1960/1909). *The Rites of Passage*. Chicago: The University of Chicago Press.

Gimbutas, M. (1989). *Language of the Goddess*. San Francisco: Harper SanFrancisco.

Good, G.E. & Wood, P.K. (1995). Male gender role conflict, depression, and help seeking: Do college men face double jeopardy? *Journal of Counseling and Development*, 74, 70–75.

Greenberg, J.R. & Mitchell, S.A. (1983). *Object Relations in Psychoanalysis*. Cambridge: Harvard Press.

Greenson, R. (1968). Dis-identifying from mother: Its special importance for the boy. *International Journal of Psycho-Analysis*, 49, 370–374.

Griffths, P.E. (1997). *What Emotions Really Are: The Problem of Psychological Categories*. Chicago: University of Chicago Press.

Hayes, J.A. & Mahalik, J.R. (2000). Gender role conflict and psychological distress in male counseling center clients. *Psychology of Men and Masculinity*, 2, 116–125.

Horney, K. (1950). *Neurosis and Human Growth: The Struggle toward Self-realization*. Norton: New York.

Izard, C.E. (1991). *The Psychology of Emotions*. New York: Plenum Press.

Johnson, R.A. (1989). *He: Understating Male Psychology*. New York: Harper Paperback.

Jaeger, C.S. (1985). *The Origins of Courtliness*. Philadelphia: University of Pennsylvania Press.

Jung, C.G. (1968). *Analytic Psychology: Its Theory and Applications*. New York: Vintage.

Kohut, H. (1984). *How Does Analysis Cure?* Chicago: The University of Chicago Press.

Klein, M. (1930). The importance of symbol-formation in the development of the ego. *International Journal of Psycho-Analysis*, 11, 24–39.

Klein, M. (1940). Mourning and its relationship to manic-depressive states. *International Journal of Psychoanalysis*, 21.

Levant, R.F. (1995). Toward reconstruction of masculinity. In W.S. Pollack & R.F. Levant (eds.), *New Psychology of Men* (pp. 229–251). New York: Basic Books.

Levant, R.F. & Pollack, W. (1995). Introduction. In W.S. Pollack & R.F. Levant (eds.), *New psychology of men* (pp.1–10). New York: Basic Books.

Levant, R.F., Good, G.E., Cook, S.W., O'Neil, J.M., Smalley, K.B., & Owen, K. (2006). The normative male alexithymia scale: Measurement of a gender-linked syndrome. *Psychology of Men and Masculinity*, 7, 212–224.

Mahalik, J.R., Cournoyer, R., DeFranc, W., Cherry, M., & Napolitano, J.M. (1998). Gender role conflict: Predictors of men's utilization of psychological defenses. *Journal of Counseling Psychology*, 45, 247–255.

Mahler, M., Pine, F., & Bergman, A. (1975). *The Psychological Birth of the Human Infant*. New York: Basic Books.

McClure, E.B. (2000). A meta-analytic review of sex differences in facial expression processing and their development in infants, children, and adolescents. *Psychological Bulletin*, 126, 424–453.

McMurtry, L. (1985). *Lonesome Dove*. New York: Simon & Schuster.

Miller, A. (1999/1949) *Death of a Salesman*. New York: Penguin.

Murstein, B. I., Cerreto, M., & MacDonald, M. G. (1977). A theory and investigation of the effect of exchange-orientation on marriage and friendship. *Journal of Marriage and the Family*, 39, 543–548.

O'Neil, J.M. (2008). Summarizing twenty-five years of research on men's gender role conflict using the gender role conflict scale: New research paradigms and clinical implications. *The Counseling Psychologist*, 36, 358–445.

O'Neil, J.M. & Egan, J. (1992b). Men's gender role transitions over the life span: Transformations and fears of femininity. *Journal of Mental Health Counseling*, 14, 305–324.

O'Neil, J.M., Helms, B., Gable, R., David, L., & Wrightsman, L. (1986). Gender role conflict scale: College men's fear of femininity. *Sex Roles*, 14, 335–350.

Pleck, J.H. (1981). *The Myth of Masculinity*. Cambridge, MA: MIT Press.

Pollack, W.S. (1999) *Real Boys: Rescuing Our Sons from the Myth of Boyhood*. New York: Henry Holt & Company.

Pope, H.G. and Olivardia, R. (1999). Evolving ideals of male body image as seen through action toys. *International Journal of Eating Disorders* 26(1), 65–72.

Rochlen, A.B., McKelley, R.A., Suizzo, M., & Scaringi, V. (2008). Predictors of relationship satisfaction, psychological well-being, and life satisfaction among stay-at-home fathers. *Psychology of Men and Masculinity*, 9(1), 17–28.

Sandler, J. & Rosenblatt, B. (1962). The concept of the representational world. *Psychoanalytic Study of the Child*, 17, 128–145.

Springsteen. B. "Secret Garden." *Secret Garden*. [sound recording]. Phantom Sound & Vision.

Terman, K. & Miles, C. (1936/1968). *Sex and Personality: Studies in Masculinity and Femininity*. New York: Russell & Russell.

Thibaut, J.W. & Kelly, H.H. (1959). *The Social Psychology of Groups*. New York: Wiley.

Thompkins, C.D. & Rando, R.A. (2003). Gender role conflict and shame in college men. *Psychology of Men and Masculinity*, 4(1), 79–81.

Turner, V. (1966). *The Ritual Process: Structure and Anti-structure*. Ithaca, New York: Scholastic Press.

Weinberg, M.K., Tronick, E.Z., Cohn, J.F., & Olson, K.L. (1999). Gender differences in emotional expressivity and self-regulation during early infancy. *Developmental Psychology*, 35, 175–188.

Williams, T. (1958). *Cat on a Hot Tin Roof*. New York: Signet.

Winnicott, D.W. (1971). *Playing and Reality*. Middlesex, England: Penguin.

Winnicott, D.W. (1958). *The Capacity To Be Alone: The Maturational Process and the Facilitating environment*. New York: International Press.

# INDEX